Handbook of Colposcopy

Second edition

Edited by

David M. Luesley
Professor of Gynaecological Oncology
Academic Department of Obstetrics and Gynaecology

Mahmood I. Shafi
Consultant Gynaecological Surgeon and Oncologist

Joseph A. Jordan
Medical Director

*Birmingham Women's Hospital
Queen Elizabeth Medical Centre
Birmingham, UK*

D1333819

ARNOLD

A member of the Hodder Headline Group
LONDON · NEW YORK · NEW DELHI

First published in Great Britain in 2002 by
Arnold, a member of the Hodder Headline Group,
338 Euston Road, London NW1 3BH

http://www.arnoldpublishers.com

Distributed in the USA by
Oxford University Press Inc.,
198 Madison Avenue, New York, NY10016
Oxford is a registered trademark of Oxford University Press

© 2002 Arnold

Whilst the advice and information in this book are believed to be true and
accurate at the date of going to press, neither the authors nor the publisher
can accept any legal responsibility or liability for any errors or omissions
that may be made. In particular (but without limiting the generality of the
preceding disclaimer) every effort has been made to check drug dosages;
however, it is still possible that errors have been missed. Furthermore,
dosage schedules are constantly being revised and new side-effects
recognized. For these reasons the reader is strongly urged to consult the
drug companies' printed instructions before administering any of the drugs
recommended in this book.

British Library Cataloguing in Publication Data
A catalogue record for this book is available from the British Library

Library of Congress Cataloging-in-Publication Data
A catalog record for this book is available from the Library of Congress

ISBN 0 340 80660 5

2 3 4 5 6 7 8 9 10

Publisher: Joanna Koster
Production Editor: James Rabson
Production Controller: Martin Kerans
Cover Design: Terry Griffiths

Typeset in 10/13pt Sabon by Cambrian Typesetters, Frimley, Surrey
Printed and bound in Malta by Gutenberg Press Ltd

What do you think about this book? Or any other Arnold title?
Please send your comments to feedback.arnold@hodder.co.uk

CONTENTS

Colour plate section appears between pages 120 and 121

CONTRIBUTORS

Dr J. Cordiner
Consultant Obstetrician and Gynaecologist, Queen Mother's Hospital, Yorkhill, Glasgow G3 8SH

Dr G.P. Downey
Consultant Obstetrician and Gynaecologist, City Hospital NHS Trust, Dudley Road, Birmingham B18 7QH

Dr I.D. Duncan
Reader in Obstetrics and Gynaecology, Ninewells Hospital and Medical School, Dundee, DDI 9SY

T. Freeman-Wang
Research Fellow, The Royal Free Hospital, Pond Street, London NW3

Mr D.A. Hicks
Consultant Physician in GU Medicine, Department of Genitourinary Medicine, Royal Hallamshire Hospital, Glossop Road, Sheffield S10 2JF

Dr J. Johnson
Consultant Histopathologist, Department of Pathology, City Hospital, Hucknall Road, Nottingham NG5 1PB

Mr J.A. Jordan
Medical Director, Birmingham Women's Hospital, Edgbaston, Birmingham B15 2TG

Professor H.C. Kitchener
Professor of Gynaecological Oncology, Academic Unit of Obstetrics and Gynaecology and Reproductive Health Care, St Mary's Hospital, Whitworth Park, Manchester M13 0JH

Mr F.G. Lawton
Consultant Gynaecological Cancer Surgeon, Department of Obstetrics and Gynaecology, King's College Hospital, Denmark Hill, London SE5 8RX

Professor D.M. Luesley
Professor of Gynaecological Oncology, Academic Department of Obstetrics and Gynaecology, Birmingham Women's Hospital, Edgbaston, Birmingham B15 2TG

Dr J. Murphy
Department of Obstetrics and Gynaecology, Blackrock Clinic, Rock Road, Co. Dublin, EIRE

Mr C.W.E. Redman
Consultant Obstetrician and Gynaecologist, Academic Department of Obstetrics and Gynaecology, North Staffordshire Hospital NHS Trust, Newcastle Road, Stoke-on-Trent ST4 6QG

Dr T.P. Rollason
Consultant Pathologist, Birmingham Women's Hospital, Edgbaston, Birmingham B15 2TG

Mr M.I. Shafi
Consultant Gynaecological Surgeon and Oncologist, Birmingham Women's Hospital, Edgbaston, Birmingham B15 2TG

Mr P. Walker
Consultant Gynaecologist, The Royal Free Hospital, Pond St, London NW3

Mr D.R. Williams
Cytopathology Department, George Eliot Hospital, Nuneaton, Warwickshire CV10 7DJ

ABBREVIATIONS

AGUS	Atypical glandular cells of uncertain significance
AIS	Adenocarcinoma-*in-situ*
ASCUS	Atypical squamous cells of uncertain significance
AW	Acetowhite
BCC	Benign cell change
BNA	Borderline nuclear abnormalities
BSCC	British Society of Cervical Cytology
BSCCP	British Society of Colposcopy and Cervical Pathology
CGIN	Cervical glandular intraepithelial neoplasia
CIN	Cervical intraepithelial neoplasia
CTZ	Congenital transformation zone
DES	Diethylstilboestrol
DLE	Diathermy loop excision
DNCB	Dinitrochlorobenzene
ECC	Endocervical curettage
ESI	Early stromal invasion (now more correctly stage Ia_1 cancer)
FHSA	Family Health Service Authority
FIGO	International Federation of Obstetrics and Gynecology
5-FU	5-Fluorouracil
GUM	Genitourinary medicine
HGCGIN	High-grade cervical glandular intraepithelial neoplasia
HGIL	High-grade glandular intraepithelial lesion
HPV	Human papillomavirus
HSIL	High-grade squamous intraepithelial lesion
HSV	Herpes simplex virus
IFCPC	International Federation of Cervical Pathology and Colposcopy
K	Koilocytes or koilocytosis
LBC	Liquid-based cytology
LEEP	Loop electrosurgical excisional procedure
LGCGIN	Low-grade cervical glandular intraepithelial neoplasia
LLETZ	Large loop excision of the transformation zone
LSIL	Low-grade squamous intraepithelial lesion
LVSI	Lymph-vascular space involvement

MIN	Multifocal intraepithelial neoplasia
NAC	National Association of Cytologists
PPV	Positive predictive value
NCN	National Co-ordinating Network
NHSCSP	National Health Service Cervical Screening Programme
PIN	Penile intraepithelial neoplasia
RCOG	Royal College of Obstetricians and Gynaecologists
SCJ	Squamocolumnar junction
SIL	Squamous intraepithelial lesion
TAH	Total abdominal hysterectomy
TV	*Trichomonas vaginalis*
TZ	Transformation zone
USIL	Ungraded squamous intraepithelial lesion
VaIN	Vaginal intraepithelial neoplasia
VIN	Vulvar intraepithelial neoplasia

chapter 1

THE NORMAL ANATOMY AND HISTOLOGY OF THE CERVIX

T.P. Rollason

GROSS ANATOMY

The cervix is the most caudal portion of the uterus, and protrudes into the upper vagina. It measures 2.5 to 3 cm in length in the adult multigravida, and makes up one-third to one-half of the length of the uterus. The cervix is demarcated from the uterine corpus by a fibromuscular junction termed the internal os, and the endocervical canal opens into the vaginal vault at the external os. The vagina is fused circumferentially to the cervix, thereby dividing it into upper, supravaginal and lower, vaginal portions. These portions are of approximately the same length. As the uterus is normally anteverted, the cervix is usually angulated downward and backward. The shape of the cervix is highly variable. The nulliparous cervix has a circular external os and a diameter of approximately 2.0–2.5 cm. The multiparous cervix is larger and more protruding and has a transverse, slit-like external os. The reflections of the vaginal epithelium around the sides of the cervix constitute the vaginal fornices. The vaginal portion of the cervix (portio vaginalis) is divided into anterior and posterior lips; the anterior is shorter and projects lower than the posterior. Both cervical lips are normally in contact with the posterior vaginal wall.

The cervical canal connects the uterine isthmus (internal os) with the external os. This is an elliptical cavity showing longitudinal ridges (plicae palmatae) composed of epithelium and connective tissue. The canal has a maximum diameter of approximately 7–8 mm and is approximately 3 cm long; it is also flattened anteroposteriorly.

The cervical stroma is made up of fibrous, muscular and elastic tissue. Fibrous tissue predominates, with smooth muscle located mainly in the endocervix and increasing in relative proportion as the internal os is approached. At the isthmus, smooth muscle and fibrous tissue are present in approximately equal proportions and in concentric arrangement, making up a functional sphincter.

Congenital abnormalities of the cervix usually result from abnormal development and fusion of the Mullerian ducts and are usually therefore seen in association with uterine body maldevelopment.

HISTOLOGY

'ORIGINAL'(NATIVE) SQUAMOUS EPITHELIUM

The vaginal portion of the cervix (ectocervix) is lined by stratified squamous epithelium, which in its normal state is not keratinized on light microscopy. This epithelium is replenished by proliferation of basal cells every 4–5 days during reproductive life. Maturation may be accelerated by oestrogen and inhibited, at the mid-zone of the epithelium, by progestagens. In adult life this epithelium is fully mature and glycogen-laden due to oestrogenic stimulation. In post-menopausal women the epithelium undergoes atrophy, with thinning, loss of differentiation and loss of glycogen; the whole epithelium then appears to consist of basal and parabasal-type cells. In the pre-menopausal female the epithelium is of similar appearance to that of the post-menopausal woman. During pregnancy, superficial maturation is lost under the influence of elevated progesterone concentrations.

It is usual to divide the ectocervical epithelium into three zones: basal; mid-zone; and superficial (Figure 1.1). The basal zone is composed of one or two layers of cylindrical or elliptical cells approximately 10 μm in diameter. These have scant cytoplasm and nuclei orientated perpendicular to the underlying basal lamina (basal membrane). The cells of this layer are actively dividing. The lower few layers of the mid-zone contain larger cells than the basal layer with more cytoplasm, often termed parabasal cells. In normal epithelium mitoses are seen in these cells as well as the basal layer, but with less frequency. Glycogen synthesis occurs in this layer. The upper midzone or intermediate cell zone is composed of

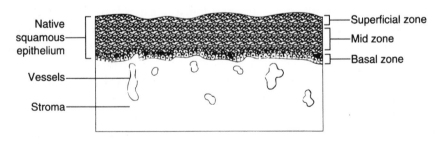

Figure 1.1 Ectocervical squamous epithelium.

non-dividing, glycogen-rich cells that show a gradual increase in cytoplasm with increasing height. The overall pattern of this zone is often termed 'basket-weave'. The cells of the superficial zone show flattening and an overall cell diameter of approximately 50 µm. The nuclei are small and pyknotic and the cytoplasm glycogen-rich and eosinophilic. The epithelial surface is cornified, and on electron microscopy a complex surface pattern of microridges is present; these are believed together to help prevent trauma to the underlying layers and stop infective agents from entering the deep epithelium. Under some exogenous stimuli keratinization occurs above the superficial cells; this is represented by a dense, eosinophilic layer of variable thickness.

The atrophic epithelium of post-menopausal women shows little or no surface epithelial maturation and absent or sparse stromal papillae (rete pegs are not normally seen even in the mature cervix).

'ORIGINAL' (NATIVE) COLUMNAR EPITHELIUM

The endocervical columnar epithelium is composed of a single layer of mucin-secreting, columnar cells. These cells have basally placed, round or oval nuclei and uniform, slightly granular cytoplasm filled with mucin droplets (Mullerian mucinous epithelium). The relative proportions of different mucins vary with the menstrual cycle. These changes in the histochemical composition of the mucins are reflected in the actual physical consistency of the mucus; at mid-cycle it is more watery, less viscous and more abundant than at other times in the cycle and it shows the capacity for 'ferning' in smears. Occasional non-secretory cells with cilia are present, resembling tubal or endometrial ciliated cells; these probably play a role in mucin movement.

On two-dimensional sections the endocervix appears to show surface epithelium and variably spaced, underlying tubular elements. Whilst the endocervical surface epithelium is often referred to as a mucosa and the tubular elements as glands, neither statement is actually true. The surface epithelium, and epithelium of the underlying structures, has no associated submucosa and is a simple epithelium, not a mucosal surface. The endocervical 'glands' are actually deep, cleft-like infoldings of the surface epithelium with numerous blind, secondary outpouchings (Figure 1.2). The epithelium of the crypts is identical to that of the surface whereas true glands have different epithelium in their ductal elements to that in their secretory portions. Although crypts have been stated to be occasionally more than 1 cm deep, the maximum depth in well-orientated sections is closer to 8 mm (mean 3.4 mm). It is usually said that the endocervical epithelium has an origin in the subcolumnar reserve cells, and that mitoses are not seen in the columnar epithelium under normal conditions.

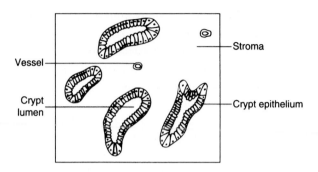

Figure 1.2 Endocervical crypts.

The endocervical epithelium, as well as crypt infolding, also shows coarse mounds or cushions called 'rugae' which are present on both lips of the cervix. This rugal pattern fuses with the longitudual 'arbor vitae' in the canal (the plicae palmatae referred to previously). There is a further fine grouping of folds to produce pendulous areas that resemble bunches of grapes.

SQUAMOUS METAPLASIA AND THE TRANSFORMATION ZONE

The squamocolumnar junction (SCJ) of the cervix is the point at which the endocervical columnar epithelium meets the ectocervical, stratified squamous epithelium (Figure 1.3). This junction is not at a fixed point on the cervix throughout life, and an understanding of the changes that occur at the SCJ throughout life is fundamental to an understanding of the processes leading up to tumour formation in the cervix.

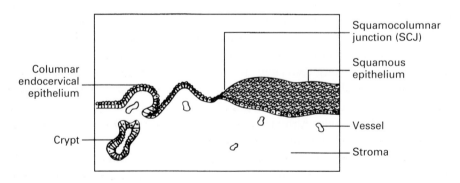

Figure 1.3 The 'original' squamocolumnar junction.

Before puberty, the SCJ is usually accepted to be located at – or close to – the external os of the cervix. This point is often called the 'original' SCJ. The junction is a sharp one. Under the influence of increasing ovarian hormones at puberty there is an increase in the size of both the corpus and cervix. This leads to eversion of the cervix which is more marked anteriorly and posteriorly than laterally, and is usually most extensive on the anterior lip. The endocervical epithelium then comes to lie on the vaginal portion of the cervix. This endocervical epithelium appears red and rough, and is often clinically termed an erosion (incorrect as no ulceration is present) or an ectopy (ectropion). This zone of eversion is most extensive in women under 20 years of age and following the first pregnancy. The everted zone, particularly when extensive, commonly takes on a papillary pattern with a chronic inflammatory cell infiltrate in the stromal cores of the papillae. This pattern is often termed papillary cervicitis but it is a physiological change, and not a true cervicitis.

The zone of eversion is exposed to the acidic environment of the vagina and it appears to be predominantly this stimulus which leads to the series of changes that follow and culminate in replacement of the everted endocervical epithelium by more resilient squamous epithelium. Two major mechanisms have in the past been favoured. The first is direct ingrowth of the adjacent squamous epithelium of the portio. Tongues of squamous epithelium grow beneath the adjacent columnar epithelium and expand between the endocervical mucinous cells and the basement membrane. The endocervical cells are gradually displaced upwards, degenerate and are sloughed. It is unclear how important a role this mechanism has, and certainly this process cannot explain the occasional presence of isolated foci of squamous metaplasia within the endocervical canal.

The second process is usually called squamous metaplasia, but it is not a truly metaplastic one, metaplasia being the replacement of one adult, differentiated epithelium by another of different type. In the first part of the process small, non-differentiated, cuboidal reserve cells, with a high nucleocytoplasmic ratio, appear beneath the columnar epithelium. These usually appear first on the upper, more exposed parts of the villous outgrowths and superficial crypts. The reserve cells proliferate to produce a layer several cells thick (reserve cell hyperplasia). At this stage the columnar cells remain as a complete or incomplete surface layer. These multilayered reserve cells then begin differentiation to clearly squamous cells with increasing amounts of eosinophilic cytoplasm, but without surface maturation and with little intracellular glycogen and a now incomplete persisting surface columnar cell layer (incomplete or immature squamous metaplasia) (Figure 1.4). Finally, all of the surface columnar cells are either shed or degenerate, and the squamous epithelium then fully matures. There is therefore now a new SCJ – the 'physiological' or 'functional' SCJ. The zone where columnar epithelium has been converted to squamous is termed the 'transformation zone' (Figure 1.5). Viewed

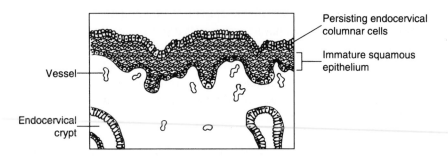

Figure 1.4 Immature squamous metaplasia.

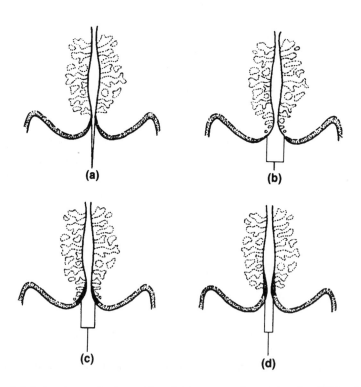

Figure 1.5 Relative changes in the position of the squamocolumnar junction (SCJ) and transformation zone as the cervix changes under endocrine influences. **(a)** Original SCJ. **(b)** New SCJ. **(c)** Transformation zone (TZ) (metaplastic squamous epithelium). **(d)** TZ inside canal. (Source: reproduced with permission from Rollason, T. P. (1995) The normal anatomy and histology of the cervix, vagina and vulva, in *Intraepithelial Neoplasia of the Female Lower Genital Tract* (eds D. Luesley, J. Jordan and R.M. Richart), Churchill Livingstone, Edinburgh, Chapter 1.)

at the end of the process of metaplasia, the transformation zone epithelium may be indistinguishable from the native ectocervical epithelium.

Apart from hormonal effects and vaginal acidity, other possible causes of metaplasia, and accelerants of the process, include inflammatory damage, chronic irritation, coitus (prostaglandin exposure) and direct trauma.

The process of metaplasia may extend into the shallower underlying crypts for their full depth and eventually obliterate them, but usually the crypts either persist, lined by endocervical epithelium, or are partly lined by squamous cells. That the surface epithelium is metaplastic may therefore be deduced from the presence of underlying crypts, as there is very little overlapping of crypts by 'original' squamous surface cells. The openings of the crypts may still be evident on the cervical surface of the transformation zone, but the squamous proliferation may lead to their blockage; this produces the very common 'Nabothian follicles'. These are in reality mucus retention cysts of the crypts due to continued mucin production, with cystic dilatation related to lack of mucin drainage. The cysts may rupture leading to a local macrophage response, sometimes with associated inflammation and fibrosis. If the crypts become completely separated from the surface epithelium after the crypt epithelium has undergone replacement by squamous cells, then a squamous inclusion cyst may develop.

Whilst, as previously indicated, cervical eversion and thus squamous metaplasia are most marked during adolescence and pregnancy, the process continues throughout adult life, and all stages of the processes described above are commonly seen in cervical biopsy specimens. After the menopause, the shrinkage of the cervical stroma causes 'retraction' of the SCJ into the endocervical canal. The process of squamous metaplasia is not a reversible one, and the canal is then lined in its lower portion by squamous epithelium.

THE CONGENITAL TRANSFORMATION ZONE (CTZ)

The CTZ is essentially a zone where endocervical epithelium has undergone squamous metaplasia in late intrauterine or early extrauterine life. It may be related to metaplasia in a zone of endocervical epithelium, which passed onto the portio under the influence of maternal oestrogen and was replaced by squamous epithelium when the oestrogenic stimulus declined. Alternatively, it may be that the CTZ is formed in a similar manner to essentially identical zones seen in DES exposed women, i.e. due to incomplete conversion of the early cuboidal epithelium of the vaginal angle at the upper (uterine) end to squamous epithelium, followed by gradual squamous replacement in late intrauterine and extrauterine life.

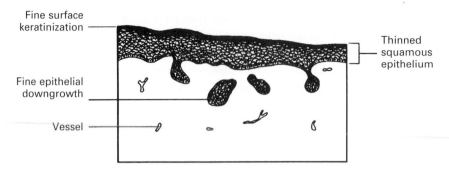

Figure 1.6 The congenital transformation zone.

The histological features of the CTZ in a typical case are: a thinned epithelium with shallow, fine (but blunt-ended) epithelial downgrowths, low or absent epithelial glycogen, and a very fine layer of surface keratinization (Figure 1.6). The epithelium gives the impression of being immature in its lower half, but maturing abnormally rapidly to keratinization over a few cell layers. The junction with the 'normal' ectocervical squamous epithelium is usually tangential but sharp and, when seen in the adult, a zone of more typical 'adult' type squamous metaplasia usually separates the CTZ from the SCJ. The low glycogen, thin epithelium, etc. may lead to a mistaken colposcopic impression of cervical intraepithelial neoplasia (CIN).

CERVICAL CHANGES DURING PREGNANCY

Under the stimulus of gestational hormones the cervix softens and enlarges. This is due to increased vascularity and stromal oedema. Acute inflammatory changes are also commonly seen in the superficial stroma. In late pregnancy there is accumulation of large amounts of extracellular glycoprotein and collagen disruption leading to further softening, facilitating dilatation, etc. in labour. Decidualization of the stroma under progestational effects is common in the superficial stroma. It may be patchy or diffuse and affects both endocervix and the ectocervix. Some degree of decidualization occurs in more than one-third of pregnant women, and takes some weeks to disappear after delivery. Occasionally, an Arias-Stella reaction may also be seen in endocervical epithelium in pregnancy.

Macroscopically, decidual foci appear as raised vascular nodules, and colposcopically they may closely resemble invasive carcinoma. Very occasionally foci of decidualization may be seen in the absence of pregnancy or obvious endometriosis; usually in association with progestagen therapy. As indicated previously, very extensive zones of cervical 'erosion' are classically seen in pregnancy, and immature metaplasia and reserve cell hyperplasia are extensive. This is most striking in primigravidae. There are probably two major processes underlying the epithelial changes seen: the first is the eversion of the endocervical canal epithelium; and the second is gaping of the os. These changes are more marked in first pregnancy, and tend to occur later in pregnancy in multiparous women.

LEARNING POINTS

- **Ectocervical epithelium**: this is stratified squamous epithelium and repopulates every 5 days. Oestrogen shortens the repopulation time. In the elderly, atrophy occurs and differentiation is reduced, making cytological and histological interpretation difficult.
- **Endocervical epithelium**: this is a columnar, mucinous Mullerian epithelium. Branching epithelial downgrowths are present producing crypts. These are not true glands.
- **Squamocolumnar junction (SCJ)**: this is the border between the squamous ectocervical epithelium and the endocervical columnar epithelium. The 'original' SCJ is where the 'native' epithelium met the endocervical epithelium in childhood. The 'physiological' SCJ is where the SCJ is seen after the effects of endogenous and exogenous hormones, pregnancy, etc.
- **Transformation zone**: the area where the native endocervical epithelium has been converted to squamous epithelium. This new squamous epithelium covers endocervical crypts, and the crypt openings may be still present or the crypts represented by spherical surface humps 2–4 mm in diameter. Nabothian follicles are mucus retention cysts formed by the blockage of the crypt neck by the squamous overgrowth.
- **Squamous metaplasia**: alteration of the endocervical columnar epithelium into squamous epithelium. It occurs via a stage of undifferentiated reserve cell growth (reserve cell hyperplasia) followed by squamous differentiation. Immature metaplasia is the stage at which there is squamous replacement, but with retention of surface endocervical columnar cells. Laser therapy, trauma, etc. speeds up the metaplastic process.
- **Congenital transformation zone (CTZ)**: in intrauterine or early post-uterine life, changes in the hormonal profile lead to the formation of a limited transformation zone of different pattern to that in the adult. This persists into

adult life and shows low epithelial glycogen content, fine surface keratinization and fine epithelial downgrowths.

- **Ectopy** or **erosion**: in reproductive life columnar epithelium is seen on the ectocervical surface to some extent, this is often clinically referred to as an ectopy or erosion. It is usually more extensive on the anterior lip. The formation of such endocervical covered zones is stimulated by oestrogen, progestagens and, particularly, pregnancy after which they may persist for some years. Papillary cervicitis (papillary ectropion) is simply a variant of this pattern.
- **Decidualization**: In pregnancy, both focal and diffuse decidualization of the cervical stroma may occur. This change is associated with increased vascularization and oedema and may be mistaken clinically for malignancy.

MCQs

For answers to Questions, see Appendix C.

1. **The ectocervical native epithelium is:**
    a. Of columnar mucinous type.
    b. Resistant to hormone effects.
    c. Of multilayered squamous type.
    d. Commonly ulcerated.
    e. Very fragile in comparison to the endocervical epithelium.

2. **The 'physiological' squamocolumnar junction:**
    a. Is where the squamous and endocervical epithelium met in childhood.
    b. Is a fixed point.
    c. Moves under the influence of hormones.
    d. Is usually well within the endocervical canal in the pre-menopausal woman.
    e. Does not exist.

3. **The transformation zone:**
    a. Is where native endocervical epithelium has been converted to squamous epithelium.
    b. Is no longer present in post-menopausal women.
    c. Never has underlying crypts.
    d. Never contains crypt openings.

4. **Squamous metaplasia is not:**
   a. A physiological process.
   b. Brought about by the effect of vaginal acidity.
   c. Stimulated by trauma.
   d. Caused by human papillomaviruses.
   e. Preceded by reserve cell hyperplasia.

5. **The congenital transformation zone is:**
   a. Formed post-menopausally.
   b. Related to uterine fundal abnormalities.
   c. Formed in pre-natal or early post-natal life.
   d. Often associated with excess epithelial glycogen production.
   e. Invisible colposcopically.

chapter 2

CERVICAL CYTOLOGY

D. R. Williams

HISTORY AND INTRODUCTION

The first illustrations of shed cells from tumours as seen under a microscope were published 150 years ago. These early observations were followed during the next 50 years by descriptions of cells from sputum, urine, cerebrospinal fluid, gastric washings and lymph node aspirates.

Babes in Bucharest, and Papanicolaou in New York introduced diagnostic cytology of the female genital tract almost simultaneously, in 1928. However, neither of these seminal observations made any major clinical impact, and it was not until Papanicolaou and Traut's later published works on uterine cancer detection in the 1940s that any momentum was gained. Today, five decades after the publication of Papanicolaou's Atlas, and countless debates on the merits of cytological diagnosis in gynaecology, it is generally considered that the cervical smear is one of the most effective health tools ever introduced. There is also little doubt that its effectiveness has been considerably improved over the past 20 years by the increasing use of colposcopy. The combination of smear and colposcope provides a very potent weapon in the quest to reduce deaths from cervical cancer.

FALSE-NEGATIVE RESULTS: CAUSES AND IMPLICATONS FOR SCREENING

The prime concern is to detect those women with significant degrees of pre-cancer, and to prevent progression to invasive disease by destruction or removal of these precursor lesions. The greatest flaw in the detection process is the potential for false-negative results. This is made more acute when, unlike diagnostic cytology from other sites where the test is only part of the overall diagnostic process, in gynaecological screening a negative test may remove the patient from medical care for three to five years. False-negative results may occur because of inadequate sampling, incorrect laboratory processing, or detection and interpretative errors of the cell samples.

It must be emphasized that cervical cytology is primarily used as a case-finding procedure for squamous precursor lesions (cervical intraepithelial neoplasia; CIN). It does not diagnose invasive lesions, nor lesions arising in endocervical tissues reliably. Aggressive tumours can rapidly utilize the available blood supply, such that the presenting surface becomes necrotic and frequently produces an inflammatory exudate only. When sampled, in the absence of relevant symptoms or suspicion on naked-eye appearance of the cervix at the time of smear taking, these smears may well be reported as non-specific inflammatory changes only – the classic 'false-negative' smear result. A clinically suspicious cervix must be biopsied, regardless of the cytology test result.

THE PROCESS OF SCREENING A CERVICAL SMEAR

It may be worthwhile to underline at this point that cytology is not the precise science some would wish it to be, but more an acquired artform. Schenk likens the process of searching for an abnormal cell to "detecting large cars among smaller cars while flying 1000 metres high in an area 230 kilometres in length and 720 metres broad within five minutes at a velocity of twice the speed of sound". Primary screeners rely heavily on experience for building up a mental database of case recognition features. This database is reinforced by comparisons of cytological predictions versus final histological outcome. The frequency of encountering these features is a major factor in adding weight to likelihood of underlying pathology. This cannot be 'taught' easily with conventional demonstration/response training routines. Intensive exposure to archival rarities frequently results in overcalling and a subsequent lack of trust by the clinical team. So, while practical exposure to common cytological categories of cervical disease is essential, and with experience reliably uniform, cytological encounters with rare disease states are frequently overlooked, screening omissions being revealed with clinical presentation and subsequent biopsy. However, careful observation and audit of practise with continuing input from accumulated knowledge should maintain reasonable accuracy of detection, and minimize false negatives (sensitivity) and false positives (specificity).

Recently, the problem of screener performance has been addressed by the adoption of rapid rescreening of all negative smears, the proscription of sensible targets and standards for service provision, and the participation in external quality assurance schemes by all laboratories working in the National Health Service Cervical Screening Programme (NHSCSP). In addition, the initial publication and recent revision of the NHSCSP's *Achievable Standards, Benchmarks for Reporting, and Criteria for Evaluating Cervical Cytopathology* has enhanced screening performance considerably. All screening laboratories are now obliged to collect and report an array of performance outcome measures, which are monitored both internally and regionally, and published annually in the DOH Statistical Review. Centrally funded and regionally organized QA external inspections, along the lines of the highly successful model employed for breast cancer screening, ensure constant vigilance for any cracks appearing in the system.

HOW TO TAKE AND PREPARE SMEARS

The accuracy of the cytological examination of a cervical smear depends predominantly on the quality of the material collected, and the preparation and staining thereafter. Doctors or nurses taking the smear must be fully aware of the purpose and principles of the screening programme, and ideally have attended a recommended course of instruction in smear taking and counselling.

INSTRUMENTS FOR TAKING A SMEAR

There are currently a variety of samplers available for smear taking both from the cervix and the endocervical canal. It must be emphasized that endocervical brush sampling is not a part of routine screening, but may be useful in taking smears post-treatment or perhaps when an endocervical lesion is suspected. If other non-standard techniques are employed, then this should be clearly stated on the request form. Not all laboratories are experienced in the differing appearances from these samplers and high pick-up of minor cytological abnormalities, poor discrimination between reactive and neoplastic appearances and a high number of inadequate samples may follow (Figure 2.1).

Ayre and Aylesbury spatulas
Most smears will be taken with a standard Ayres spatula or the modified Aylesbury version. In any event, the most important feature is in the application and use of the sampler and not the particular shape or design.

The aim of the smear is to sample the whole of the transformation zone (TZ) (the squamocolumnar junction; SCJ) which should be achieved with a full 360-degree sweep, first clockwise then anti-clockwise with the blade of the spatula

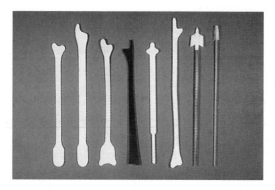

Figure 2.1 Commercially available sampling devices.

firmly applied to the cervix. If on the first sweep bleeding occurs, the spatula should be withdrawn and the cells obtained with the initial sweep spread and fixed immediately.

If the TZ is on the outer aspect of the ectocervix, this should be sampled, after the usual rotational cell collection, with firm diagonal sweeps encompassing the apparent SCJ.

If there is blood or purulent mucus covering the os, this should be gently pushed aside by the sampler before the smear is taken. Generalized swabbing is not recommended, as diagnostic cells may be lost.

When sampling a dry, atrophic cervix, it is recommended that the spatula be dampened with normal saline to help cell recovery and minimize any drying artefact.

Cervex brush

The technique using the cervex brush is similar, but the bristles are D-shaped and their cutting edge is designed to work in a clockwise fashion. With the long bristles introduced into the os, the brush should be rotated clockwise five times with the short bristles applied more closely to the ectocervix.

Cytobrush, Axibrush, etc: endocervical brush samplers

Endocervical samples should always be paired with ectocervical smears to achieve adequate TZ sampling. The endocervical brush should be introduced into the canal until just the last row of bristles are just visible at the external os, and then rotated through 180 degrees only. If the brush head is advanced too far into the canal, endometrial sampling may be achieved, causing possible confusion to the cytologist.

Owing to the tendency of this device to cause bleeding, ectocervical sampling should always precede endocervical collection.

MAKING THE SLIDE

The aim is to produce an even thin film across the whole surface of the glass slide, which should be clearly pre-labelled with patient surname and date of birth in pencil on the frosted end.

Both sides of the sampler should be spread swiftly and deliberately onto the slide on the same side as the frosted label. Straight neat strokes are preferred.

If an endocervical brush sample is taken, the cells should be rolled onto the slide with a firm rolling motion. Ecto- and endo-cervical samples taken at the same visit may be spread onto a single slide, but if this is done the samples must be spread side-by-side and not superimposed. The endocervical brush sample should be spread second, as it has a greater tendency to air-dry than spatula-collected samples, and the laboratory must be informed so that a longer coverslip may be used.

FIXATION

Once the cells are removed they must be preserved immediately. Alcohol is the fixative of choice, and is usually supplied in small pots, dropper bottles or aerosol sprays. Fixation must be within 30 s of spreading, as air-drying causes severe loss of nuclear detail that often renders the smear unreliable.

NEW TECHNOLOGIES

LIQUID-BASED CYTOLOGY (LBC) TECHNIQUES

The evidence for benefits accruing from adoption of LBC for routine cervical screening comes mainly from North America, where it is the FDA-approved method of choice. The technique has only recently merited serious consideration from Central Government in the UK. The Department of Health, in conjunction with the National Institute of Clinical Excellence (NICE), have directed three first-phase pilot sites to undertake feasibility studies to determine the logistics of the introduction of LBC and human papillomavirus (HPV) triage to current practice in UK laboratories.

LBC involves making a suspension of cells from the cervical scrape sample, and this is used to produce a thin layer of cells on a slide via negative pressure and a specialized filter procedure. This also reduces obscuring elements such as polymorphs and blood, making interpretation easier.

The added cost of LBC will be over and above the considerable costs already borne by the screening service; however, there may be a payback from a limited number of economies in other areas of service provision. Savings will certainly be found by the almost total elimination of smear inadequacy (now running at some 9.8% of all UK smears for 1999–2000, or 281 000 smears in whole numbers for that period), but it would be deceptive to imagine that these will balance out completely. The benefits to UK laboratories are more likely to be measured in terms of increased overall sensitivity, less equivocation in the low-grade diagnostic spectrum, leading to less referrals for colposcopy; and savings in time and manpower reduction in smear interpretation.

JUDGING THE ACCURACY OF THE SMEAR

It is the responsibility of the smear taker to ensure that the whole of the TZ has been adequately sampled. It is not possible for the laboratory to be certain that the full circumference of the cervix has been sampled, whatever the cellularity or cell content of the smear. A smear taken from half the cervix would look the same as one from the whole circumference.

The laboratory can provide information on the cervical smear report as to whether or not there are indicators of probable TZ sampling, but this is now considered to be only useful for improved communication between laboratory and smear takers. The latest Guidelines for Achievable Standards document states "It is logical to regard cellular evidence of TZ sampling as relevant for a test in which smear takers are expected to sample that specific anatomical site. However, there is evidence of inconsistency in reporting the presence or absence of endocervical cells, and to an even greater extent, immature metaplastic cells, limiting its use as a criterion for audit". In the light of the recent upsurge in litigation however, some laboratories are requesting a written comment from smear takers on TZ sighting, and the subsequent likelihood of sampling success, as part of the minimum data set on the request form.

SMEAR REPORTS

NEGATIVE AND INFLAMMATORY SMEARS

No smear should be reported as negative unless it has a sufficient quantity of squamous cells, taking into account the woman's age and hormonal status.

A wide range of benign reactive changes may be seen in cervical cells, particularly in metaplastic cells. Inflammation of the cervix is common but, with experience, the epithelial cell changes associated with acute and chronic inflammation and repair processes can usually be distinguished from neoplasia.

Trichomonas vaginalis, *Candida*, *Actinomyces*-like organisms, bacteria and herpes simplex cytopathic effects may all be present in routine smears. These features should be reported as negative with normal recommendation for recall. There is no indication for the recommendation of an early repeat in such smears just because they harbour an infection and minor degree of inflammatory reaction. If dyskaryosis has been eliminated, these changes should be passed without comment.

INADEQUATE SMEARS

Smears are reported as inadequate in the following circumstances, if:

1. The smear is too thick, but the presence of blood and/or leukocytes in large numbers with or without any recognizable treatable condition (TV, herpes, *Candida*, *Actinomyces*, atrophy) does not necessarily make a smear inadequate, provided that the material is well spread and extra care is taken in examining the material.
2. The smear contains too few cells for an opinion, bearing in mind that the atrophic cervix will yield very few cells and that drying artefacts may be commonly encountered as a consequence.
3. Smears consist entirely of endocervical cells – a particular consequence of direct endocervical sampling.
4. Smears are poorly fixed or air-dried to the degree that assessment is impossible.

An acceptable range of smears falling within this category would be between 5.8 and 12.9%.

BORDERLINE NUCLEAR ABNORMALITIES

Inevitably, as with any subjective process, there will be grey areas when cellular changes differentiating benign atypia from early dyskaryosis are not cut-and-dried. The British Society of Cervical Cytology (BSCC) introduced the term 'borderline nuclear abnormalities' (BNA) to be used in such cases, while the international cytological community favours the acronyms described in The Bethesda System (TBS), viz. ASCUS (atypical squamous cells of uncertain significance), and AGUS (atypical glandular cells of uncertain significance).

COMPARISON OF BSCC AND BETHESDA SYSTEMS

Although the BSCC and NHSCSP does not recommend the use of The Bethesda System (TBS) for reporting cervical/vaginal smears, and continues to recommend the use of the term dyskaryosis, they do recognize similarities between that system and the classification used in the United Kingdom. The present guidelines focus on a more direct correlation between TBS and BSCC/NHSCSP terminology to allow comparison between studies using different systems, which recognize similar narrow categories within their broad categories. Differences in percentages for abnormal categories reported with the BSCC terminology and TBS may relate to differences between populations screened, screening intervals, and referral/treatment patterns, and not reflect differing standards of practice.

The BSCC and Bethesda systems are compared and contrasted in Table 2.1, which is taken from Herbert, A., Johnson, J., Patnick, J. *et al.* (1995) Achievable standards, benchmark for reporting, criteria for evaluating cervical cytopathology, in *Cytopathology* 6, Suppl. 2, 27.

Table 2.1 Comparison of the BSCC and Bethesda reporting systems for cervical/vaginal smears

	BSCC		Bethesda	
	Negative		Negative	
			BCC	
*	Borderline		ASCUS	†
			AGUS	3%
5.5%	HPV			
			HPV/LSIL	
	Mild		USIL	2%
	(ungraded)			
	Moderate			
1.6%	Severe		HSIL	
	?glandular		HGIL	0.5%
	?invasive		Cancer	

*Working party targets
†CAP Q-probe study
AGUS = Atypical glandular cells of uncertain significance
ASCUS = Atypical squamous cells of uncertain significance
BCC = Benign cell change
HGIL = High-grade glandular intraepithelial lesion
HSIL = High-grade squamous intraepithelial lesion
LSIL = Low-grade squamous intraepithelial lesion
USIL = Ungraded squamous intraepithelial lesion

There are two broad situations when the 'borderline' category is invoked. The commonest – and often least clinically significant – is when drawing the fine diagnostic line between HPV change and mild dyskaryosis. The second situation covers a diverse group of conditions in which it may be difficult to distinguish benign, reactive or reparative changes from significant degrees of dyskaryosis, or even invasive cancer on occasions.

Endocervical cells may also exhibit equivocal nuclear changes, which require considerable diagnostic experience and skill to determine their significance. Great caution should be exercised in dealing with this category, with repeat smears recommended after a maximum of 6 months and no more than once before colposcopic referral. Failure to observe this simple advice has frequently led to the subsequent development of an advanced invasive endocervical cancer, presenting following the 'minimally abnormal endocervical' index smear inadequately followed-up or ignored. Unfortunately, this situation is almost as well known to the legal profession as to our own of late.

The likelihood of spontaneous regression in the vast majority of cases of borderline nuclear change is the rationale for its management by follow-up in the first instance; moreover, the risk of the presence of CIN3 in a small percentage of these women is the rationale for investigation if the cytological changes persist.

An achievable standard range for borderline and mildly dyskaryotic smears is 4.1 to 9.5%.

DYSKARYOSIS

Dyskaryosis is the cytological nuclear change associated with a histological diagnosis of CIN. Correlation of mild moderate and severe dyskaryosis with CIN1, 2 and 3 is not exact, but moderate dyskaryosis or worse usually indicates at least underlying CIN2 (Figures 2.2 and 2.3). Mild dyskaryosis usually corresponds with CIN1, but there may be small areas of CIN2 or 3 on the same cervix. Thus, the cytological degree of dyskaryosis should be taken to indicate the minimum degree of CIN. The terminology and definitions of CIN are described in more detail in Chapter 3, whilst the comparisons and links with The Bethesda System are addressed at the end of this chapter.

- **Dyskaryosis** may be associated with HPV change, but the presence of HPV change should not affect the recommendations for management, which should only be based on the degree of dyskaryosis.
- **Mild dyskaryosis** should be an indication for referral on its second occurrence.

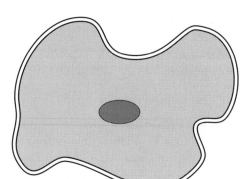

Figure 2.2 Diagrammatic representation of a normal squamous cell as determined by the relationship between nuclear and cytoplasmic area.

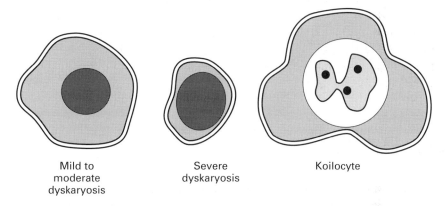

Mild to
moderate
dyskaryosis

Severe
dyskaryosis

Koilocyte

Figure 2.3 Diagrammatic representation of dyskaryotic cells demonstrating an increased nuclear/cytoplasmic ratio.

- **Moderate dyskaryosis** is very subjective and impossible to define – its severity lies somewhere between mild and severe dyskaryosis! Dyskaryotic cells that are difficult to grade (usually because of their scarcity in the smear) will usually be coded and managed as for moderate dyskaryosis. This is particularly important in recurrence of CIN after treatment, when abnormal cells may be few in number. HPV changes will also confound opinion.
- **Severe dyskaryosis** is usually seen in cells with abnormal cytoplasmic maturation and a high nuclear/cytoplasmic ratio. However, it may also occur with

intracytoplasmic keratinization, which should not be mistaken for HPV change. Moderate (including ungraded) dyskaryosis, severe dyskaryosis, ?invasive and ?glandular neoplasia, are all indications for gynaecological referral on their first occurrence.

Smears showing severe dyskaryosis in which there is tumour diathesis may be reported as suggesting cytological evidence of invasion.

Dyskaryotic cells with cytological features suggesting cervical glandular intraepithelial neoplasia (CGIN) or invasive endocervical adenocarcinoma, endometrial adenocarcinoma or extrauterine adenocarcinoma should be reported as '?glandular neoplasia'. The report usually rests on the recognition of abnormal architecture in the cell groups. Invasive endocervical adenocarcinoma usually shows the above abnormalities, and dyskaryosis is usually obvious. Smears reported thus should be referred for colposcopy with some urgency.

The achievable standard range for moderate/severe dyskaryosis is 1.0–2.0%.

TERMINOLOGY: EXTRACTS FROM NHSCSP/BSCC PUBLICATIONS

"It is axiomatic that cytology reports are not only scientifically accurate but also easily understood so that the patient receives appropriate management and advice."

"The cytology report on abnormal findings should consist of a precise description of cells in precisely defined and generally accepted cytological terms. This may be followed, if appropriate, by a prediction of the histological condition based on the overall picture, and should include a recommendation for the further management of the patient. For this reason the smear report is considered a medical consultation."

"When a prediction of histology is included as a supplementary statement to a description of the cytology, use of the terminology 'cervical intraepithelial neoplasia (CIN)' is preferred. It has the advantage of relating the histological report more clearly to the prognosis and management, than the artificial separation implied by classification into dysplasia and carcinoma in situ. Caution is advised however in the firm prediction of CIN3 because the cytologist cannot reliably exclude a microinvasive or invasive lesion."

The histological prediction is more accurately recorded on the National Cytology Form, HMR101/5 (1982), where 'severe dysplasia or carcinoma in situ (CIN3)' or 'carcinoma in situ (CIN3) or ?invasive carcinoma' are the alternatives provided.

The outcome measure for 'cytology versus histological' outcome is defined as the Positive Predictive value (PPV), and all laboratories are now required to provide a breakdown of performance against this standard. Predictive value gives a measure of the specificity of a laboratory, but not the sensitivity.

The sensitivity, specificity, predictive value and accuracy of cervical cytology is difficult – if not impossible – to calculate with accuracy, because there may be progression or regression of the lesion in the period between cytology and histology; biopsy samples may not be representative of the lesion, and the histological result is also subject to observer variation. Furthermore, the outcome of a negative test may not be known for several years after the smear was taken, by which time lesions on the cervix may have developed *de novo*, progressed or regressed.

An achievable standard depends on the laboratory obtaining results of all biopsies taken as a result of abnormal smears reported in their laboratory. Falling below the expected PPV may not result from inaccurate cytology reporting, and should be audited alongside correlation of colposcopy and biopsy findings and of histology findings in punch and excision biopsies. However, it may indicate over-calling by the laboratory. A PPV above the indicated range may be due to a high laboratory threshold for referring women for colposcopy.

The standard range for PPV for smears graded 'moderate dyskaryosis or worse' is given as 65–90%.

SCREENING PROGRAMME GUIDELINES AND OUTCOMES

The White Paper *The Health of the Nation* set a national target to reduce the mortality of cervical cancer by at least 20% by the year 2000 (from 15 per 100,000 population in 1986 to no more than 12 per 100,000, directly standardized against the European population). The NHS Cervical Screening Programme exceeded the target by the year 1997, when the rate fell to 8.9 per 100,000. It continues to fall.

This reduction has been achieved through regular screening of women aged 20–64 years, enabling prompt treatment of conditions that otherwise would have had a significant risk of development into cervical cancer. The target that at least 80% of women aged 20–64 should have had a smear within five years has been exceeded for the past four years (1997–2000).

It is essential that all 'abnormal' smears be followed-up. Guidelines on fail-safe mechanisms for the follow-up of cervical smears are published by the NHS Cervical Screening Programme National Co-ordinating Network (ed. I. D. Duncan, Oxford, 1992). The number of 'abnormal smears' has been stable over the same period of four years (between 8.1 and 8.3% of the 3,500,000 million smears (approximately) taken annually in England and Wales). The proportion of smears reported as 'moderate dyskaryosis or worse' has also remained stable at 1.6%. This represents nearly 70,000 cases per annum.

The original guidelines also set out to:

- provide acceptable and effective investigations and treatment with minimal physical or psychological side effects;
- inform women how they can reduce the risk of CIN;
- involve women both individually and collectively in the development of the programme;
- minimize the adverse effects of screening, namely anxiety and unnecessary investigations;
- make the best use of available resources for the benefit of the population at risk;
- help those working in the programme to improve their competence and find fulfilment in their work; and
- evaluate the programme and seek continual improvements in quality.

The first point has been the goal of the British Society of Colposcopy and Cervical Pathology ever since its inception, and will always be vigorously pursued.

The debate on patient involvement and access to advice and truthful information regarding the pre-cancer screening/treatment conundrum – what has been termed 'Informed consent' by some experts – has been the subject of continuing and ongoing debate within the professions.

INFORMED CONSENT

INTRODUCTION

The General Medical Council and the UKCC have both produced guidelines concerning informed consent. These deal with the principles of good practice which all registered doctors and nurses are expected to follow when seeking patients' informed consent to investigations, treatment, screening and research. The GMC guidelines also apply to other staff who may be delegated these tasks, such as practice nurses, although the doctor remains responsible for ensuring that the patient has been given sufficient time and information to make an informed decision whether they wish to be screened.

WHAT IS INFORMED CONSENT?

Informed consent involves understanding the nature and purpose of the intervention; intended and unintended side effects; risks, harms and hoped for benefits; and reasonable alternatives.

INFORMED CONSENT AND SCREENING

Screening involves testing asymptomatic people with the aim of detecting disease before it is clinically apparent and life-threatening. Anyone considering whether to consent to screening should make a properly informed decision. Particular attention must be paid to ensure that the information the person wants or ought to have is identified and provided. These points should be:

- The purpose of screening.
- The likelihood of positive and negative findings and the possibility of false-positive and false-negative results.
- The uncertainties and risks attached to the screening process.

LEARNING POINTS

- It should be emphasized to all those working in the National Cervical Screening Programme, including the patient base, that the cervical smear is normally a screening test for asymptomatic women, and that a single normal smear does not rule out invasive cancer. Indeed, false-negative rates may be highest in invasive lesions. Despite this, the smear test may also be used for diagnostic purposes and may also detect other diseases, ranging from infections to other genital tract cancers.
- The sensitivity, specificity, predictive value and accuracy of cervical cytology is impossible to calculate precisely, because the histological result (the 'gold standard' by which most surveys are compared) is itself subject to observer variation, and biopsy samples may not necessarily be representative of the lesion. Furthermore, outcome of a negative test may not be known for several years after the smear was taken, by which time lesions may have developed *de novo*, progressed or regressed.

- The anxiety levels in patients requested to return for repeat smears for inadequate or borderline categories is extremely high, and these reports should only be issued after careful deliberation. They should not be driven by fear of litigation or lack of training.
- The effectiveness of the screening programme essentially depends on the identification and treatment of CIN3. This is largely achieved by the recognition of severe, and to a lesser extent moderate, dyskaryosis on cervical smears. The treatment of CIN should be explained to the women taking part in the programme as a treatment of risk and not as a treatment of disease, and that it is most effectively detected in young women in their twenties and thirties, before the decade of life in which invasive cancer most frequently presents.
- Endocervical abnormalities may be cytologically difficult to interpret, and reports suggesting endocervical lesions, however weighted, should be investigated thoroughly.
- The NHSCSP is now acknowledged to be among the best in the world. The incidence of cervical cancer has fallen more than any other cancer, that is, by 26% between 1992 and 1997. The death rate is falling by an accelerated rate of 7% per year. Cervical cancer is an increasingly uncommon disease in the UK.

MCQs

For answers to Questions, see Appendix C.

6. **With regard to cervical smear-taking and reporting:**
   a. The person taking the smear usually decides if the sample is adequate.
   b. A smear report of moderate dyskaryosis should be managed as for mild dyskaryosis.
   c. The transformation zone is difficult to sample in postmenopausal patients.
   d. Colposcopy is not indicated following a smear report of abnormal endocervical cells.
   e. Cervical cytology can reliably detect invasive squamous cell cancer.

chapter 3

CERVICAL INTRAEPITHELIAL NEOPLASIA (CIN): TERMINOLOGY AND DEFINITIONS

J. Johnson

TERMINOLOGY OF CIN

The majority of intraepithelial disease on the cervix involves the squamous epithelium, and the term cervical intraepithelial neoplasia (CIN) refers exclusively to squamous disease. Intraepithelial neoplasia does, however, also affect the glandular or columnar epithelium, at which point the term cervical glandular intraepithelial neoplasia (CGIN) is used.

In the UK, CIN is divided into three grades, 1, 2 and 3, underlying the fact that the disease process is a continuum from normality, through the grades of CIN to invasive cancer. This also allows correlation with the three grades of cytological dyskaryosis. In the United States, the Bethesda system of reporting uses just two grades of squamous intraepithelial lesion (SIL) including human papillomavirus (HPV) changes and CIN1 in low-grade SIL (LSIL) and CIN2 and CIN3 in high-grade SIL (HSIL). The disadvantages of this system include that it incorporates non-neoplastic conditions, and it also implies that the disease is a step-wise process rather than a smooth transition.

Glandular lesions are less well understood than the squamous ones, and there is no clear sequence of progression from one grade of CGIN to another, or from CGIN to adenocarcinoma. There is a less clear system of grading than for CIN; the current recommendation being that only two grades should be recognized, namely high- and low-grade CGIN.

SQUAMOUS EPITHELIAL ABNORMALITIES

The feature which distinguishes CIN from reactive conditions is the presence, throughout the epithelial thickness, of nuclear abnormality.

CIN1

In the lowest grade of CIN the nuclear abnormalities, i.e. pleomorphism, increased nuclear-cytoplasmic ratio, nuclear enlargement, stippling of nuclear chromatin, are predominantly in the lower third of the epithelium. Abnormal mitoses may be present and support the diagnosis. In the upper two-thirds of the epithelium, maturation is visible.

CIN2

Here, the maturation occupies only the upper one-third to two-thirds of the epithelium. The nuclear abnormalities are more obvious, and there is mitotic activity with abnormal mitoses being found more commonly.

CIN3

Cytoplasmic maturation may be absent, or only seen in the upper one-third of the epithelium. Nuclear abnormalities are marked, and abnormal mitoses are usually abundant.

HPV-ASSOCIATED CHANGES

In the past, it was considered that koilocytes were pathognomonic of HPV infection, but it is now recognized that other viruses might be associated with the formation of koilocytes, and that HPV infection may be present without koilocytosis. In the absence of CIN, either 'koilocytosis-only' or 'HPV-like features' (if there is also papillomatosis, parakeratosis and multinucleation) may be reported. When CIN is present, it will be graded as above.

GLANDULAR EPITHELIAL ABNORMALITIES

CGIN is often associated with CIN, and may affect the surface epithelium as well as underlying crypts. It may also be multifocal within the endocervical canal, but usually occurs at and around the squamocolumnar junction (SCJ). CGIN is recognized by both architectural and cytological features. The architectural features include crowding, branching and budding of the glands, intraluminal papillae and a cribriform pattern of crypts, though not all of these may be present in any one case (Plate 1).

Cytological features include nuclear enlargement and loss of polarity, nuclear pleomorphism, hyperchromasia and prominent nucleoli. The nuclei may be stratified rather than in a single layer as normal. There will be mitoses, some of which may be abnormal.

High-grade CGIN is diagnosed when the features are marked and the lesion is one of adenocarcinoma-*in-situ* or CGIN3. All abnormalities of lesser degree are called low-grade CGIN.

MICROINVASIVE CARCINOMA

In the UK, microinvasive carcinoma is equivalent to FIGO Stages Ia_1 and Ia_2. FIGO Stage Ia_1 includes invasive disease where the width of the lesion is up to 7 mm and the depth is 3 mm or less from the base of the epithelium of origin. Stage Ia_2 is also up to 7 mm wide, but the depth is between 3.1 and 5 mm. The presence or absence of vascular space involvement will be recorded in the histology report, but it does not alter the staging.

There are two types of microinvasion. The first type – sometimes called 'early stromal invasion' – comprises small tongues of abnormal epithelium that push into the stroma from the base of the epithelium, usually showing CIN3 or high-grade CGIN. The invading cells often show cytoplasmic maturation with eosinophilia. There is usually a reactive lymphocytic infiltrate in the stroma that appears rather looser around the epithelial bud. The depth of such lesions is less than 1 mm from the epithelium of origin. The width should be the width of the whole field of invasion. Some multifocal lesions may be seen in several blocks taken from a loop or cone biopsy, thereby exceeding the 7 mm definition of microinvasion; these should be diagnosed as Stage lb. The second type has been called a microcarcinoma and has a confluent growth pattern. The width and depth measurements are taken as above.

These terms are applied to invasive lesions of both squamous and glandular types, although early stromal invasion is unusual in glandular carcinomas. It must be remembered that treatment regimes may be different for small adenocarcinomas than those used for microinvasive squamous cell carcinomas.

EXAMINATION OF BIOPSY SPECIMENS

The diagnosis of CIN is usually made on either a colposcopically directed punch biopsy, a large loop excision specimen, or a conization specimen. Endocervical curettage specimens may also rarely be received. Occasionally, a woman with CIN may be treated by hysterectomy.

COLPOSCOPIC PUNCH BIOPSY

During the colposcopic examination, saline and acetic acid are applied to the surface of the cervix. It is important that these are applied gently, with a dabbing rather than a rubbing action, so that the fragile epithelium is not dislodged, resulting in a denuded specimen. Biopsies need to be taken after the application of acetic acid, because this identifies the location of the lesions. This does not appear to cause any problems or recognizable artefacts.

Formalin is a perfectly adequate fixative for cervical biopsies of all types. Although Bouin's solution has advantages in the rendering of nuclear detail, the hazards associated with the use of this agent, such as its greater noxiousness and the risk of explosion if it is allowed to dry out, outweigh these. An adequate colposcopic biopsy consists of surface epithelium with underlying crypts and stroma. Stromal invasion cannot be excluded by colposcopic punch biopsy but, if the biopsy is small and superficial, without underlying stroma, then obviously no comment can be made about the presence of invasion. Punch biopsies are examined at several levels to ensure that the smallest lesions are identified.

ENDOCERVICAL CURETTAGE

Endocervical curettage is widely advocated as part of the routine colposcopic evaluation in the United States for assessing the state of the epithelium in the cervical canal, but it is not used in the UK to any extent. The material produced by endocervical curettage is scanty, consisting of mucus, blood and fragments of endocervical columnar epithelium and slivers of squamous epithelium. It is unusual for a substantial amount of stroma to be present, so that usually no comment can be made about the presence or absence of invasion. Often, all that can be said is that the epithelium is atypical; it may not be possible to assess the degree of CIN or CGIN in an endocervical curettage specimen. It is important that processing is done carefully and the blocks sectioned at levels. Clearly, no attempt at orientation can be made.

LLETZ SPECIMEN AND CONE BIOPSY

The procedures of large loop excision of the transformation zone (LLETZ) and knife cone biopsy result in generally similar specimens, as does laser excision, except that in LLETZ specimens glandular epithelium at the excision margins may have 'streaming' artefacts. If a glandular lesion is being excised, a cold knife or laser cone is preferable to LLETZ excision. The excised tissue should immediately be placed in ample fixative, which is normally formalin. A marker stitch is only of value if the gynaecologist wishes to know the anteroposterior distribution of the lesions; it does not need to be done for the pathologist's benefit. The fixed conization specimen is divided into blocks by parallel sagittal cuts, each 2–3 mm apart. Wherever possible the cone should be excised in one piece so that excision of the lesion can be assessed. Epithelium may be lost if the cone is opened, and orientation is impossible if a LLETZ is received in several pieces.

HYSTERECTOMY SPECIMEN

If a woman with CIN is treated by hysterectomy, then the cervix is removed from the hysterectomy specimen and handled in the same way as a conization specimen.

LEARNING POINTS

- Cervical intraepithelial neoplasia (CIN) is a spectrum of disease, with no clearly defined diagnostic boundaries within the spectrum or at its lower end, where it merges with physiological changes.
- There is disagreement as to whether CIN should be classified by division into three or two grades and whether human papillomavirus (HPV) infection should be included with CIN.
- Increasing grades of severity of CIN show increasing thickness of undifferentiated cells in the epithelium, increasing nuclear abnormalities and an increasing number of mitotic figures. Abnormal mitotic figures are more obvious in the more severe grades, but may be seen in CIN1.
- CGIN and progression to adenocarcinoma is less well understood than the natural history of squamous disease.
- The earliest stages of invasion are seen as breaks in the basement membrane, with buds of squamous cells pushing into the stroma.
- Slightly more advanced but still very small preclinical carcinomas (microcarcinomas) are assessed by measurement in two dimensions: the greatest depth

of invasion and the widest lateral spread. These measurements are used to guide management, which may be different for squamous and adenocarcinomas at the same stage.
- Punch biopsies should be examined at several levels.
- Invasion cannot be excluded on punch biopsies.
- Excision specimens (LLETZ and cone biopsies) are serially blocked at 2.0–3.0 mm intervals and entirely embedded. They should not be opened before fixation.
- Knife cone biopsies are preferred for excision of glandular lesions.

MCQs

For answers to Questions, see Appendix C.

7. **The following histological features distinguish CIN3 from CIN1:**
   a. CIN3 shows greater nuclear pleomorphism than CIN1.
   b. CIN3 shows greater variation in nuclear size than CIN1.
   c. CIN3 shows better differentiation than CIN1.
   d. Nuclei at the surface are normal in CIN1.
   e. Nucleoli are more prominent in CIN1 than in CIN3.

8. **Which of the following statements about CGIN are true?**
   a. CGIN naturally falls into three categories.
   b. The term high-grade CGIN includes adenocarcinoma-*in-situ*.
   c. There is a clear progression from low-grade CGIN to adenocarcinoma.
   d. Cervical crypts may be involved by all grades of CGIN.
   e. CGIN is best excised using LLETZ.

9. **The following are histological features of early invasive carcinoma:**
   a. Focal lymphocytic infiltrate in the stroma.
   b. Anaplasia of the invasive cells.
   c. Eosinophilia of the invasive cells.
   d. Ulceration of the surface epithelium.
   e. Focal condensation of stromal collagen.

chapter 4

THE COLPOSCOPE AND TECHNIQUES OF COLPOSCOPY

M.I. Shafi and J.A. Jordan

HISTORY AND INTRODUCTION

The colposcope is a system that allows both magnification and illumination of the cervix, and was first introduced in 1925 by Hans Hinselmann. The primary objective was to diagnose cervical cancer at its earliest stage. The magnification range is usually between 6- and 40-fold. Colposcopy was not taken up by English-speaking countries until the 1960s – approximately 20 years after the introduction of the Papanicolaou smear. However, it is important that the colposcopist is fully conversant with both cervical cytology and histopathology in order to appreciate fully the scientific basis of colposcopic appearances.

BASIC PRINCIPLES

Although several types of colposcope are available, all are based on similar principles. The major advances since the instrument's introduction have been in the light source, fibreoptic cabling and refinement of the optical systems. The colposcope is usually mounted on a freely movable stand, but can also be fixed to the examination table or wall if desired. The focal length varies between 200 and 300 mm, and this allows the colposcopist to conduct an examination in comfort. Attachments to the colposcope may include a monocular teaching arm, a video camera and a green filter. This green filter allows better definition of vascular architecture by absorbing red light so that the blood vessels appear black and prominent.

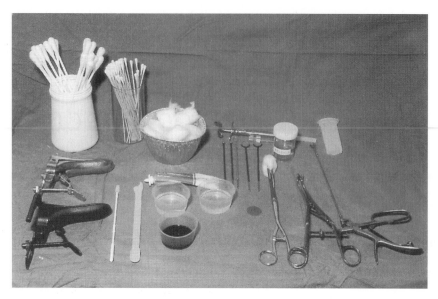

Figure 4.1 Colposcopy instrument trolley.

BASIC EQUIPMENT (Figure 4.1)

A **colposcopy couch** is preferable, as this allows the patient to be examined in a modified lithotomy position. Either the feet are placed in heel rests, or knee rests are used to support the legs. The newer hydraulic couches allow an examination position to be found easily, without discomfort to either the patient or colposcopist. A chair that can be moved up or down is advantageous for the colposcopist, again allowing the optimal examination position to be found.

Instruments should be readily to hand and placed on a nearby trolley. These should include:

- Bivalve speculum – varying sizes should be available, but the largest speculum that can comfortably be inserted should be used. Each speculum should be available with a suction tube.
- Cotton wool balls.
- Sponge-holding forceps to hold the cotton wool balls.
- Cotton-tip ('Q-tips') and jumbo swabs.
- Endocervical specula – these are useful for examination of the lower endocervical canal.

- Iris hooks, which may be used to manipulate the cervix; a skin hook may be used as a substitute.
- Biopsy forceps – a variety should be available and should be regularly sharpened.
- Three small galley pots – these are used to hold normal saline, acetic acid (3% or 5%) and Lugol's iodine.
- Endocervical curette.
- A variety of loops for use with electrosurgical equipment – these can be used both for biopsy and also for therapeutic purposes.

EXAMINATION PROCEDURE

All patients should be examined in warm surroundings and be fully informed about the procedure. Once the patient is comfortable on the examination couch, the cervix is exposed with a bivalve speculum. The cervix and upper vagina are examined at low magnification. If a cervical smear is required, then it should be performed at this stage. Care should be taken to minimize bleeding associated with smear-taking as this may confuse the subsequent assessment. Excess mucus is gently removed from the cervix with a dry or saline-soaked cotton wool ball, and the cervix is re-inspected.

Acetic acid (3% or 5%) is gently applied to the cervix and upper vagina with either a cotton wool ball or a jumbo swab, or by using a spray. The acetic acid is left *in situ* for 5–10 s; any remaining mucus is relatively easy to remove at this stage. The acetic acid will cause the columnar epithelium and abnormal epithelium to appear as white (acetowhite); this is easily distinguishable from the normal, pink squamous epithelium. If the effect of the acetic acid wears off (usually within 1 min), then the acid may be re-applied. This is important, especially if a permanent record is to be made either using colpophotographs or cervicographs of the abnormality.

Lugol's iodine may be used to outline atypical epithelium as this contains little or no glycogen and therefore will not take up the stain. Normal epithelium, conversely, is glycogen-rich and on application of Lugol's iodine will turn a dark brown colour. Columnar epithelium also contains little or no glycogen and fails to take up the stain. This test (Schiller's test) is particularly useful for colposcopists who are learning the technique, and allows minor degrees of abnormality to be detected which may otherwise have been missed. One area of confusion is that immature metaplasia or congenital transformation zones will also not take up the stain, and this may lead to a false-positive result. It is important that these situations are recognized as they are variants of normality.

Some colposcopists will use saline initially, before the application of acetic acid. This technique is particularly useful for the study of angioarchitecture but interpretation of the findings requires considerable skill.

DIGITAL IMAGING COLPOSCOPY

With the advent of digital technology, it has been possible to undertake the colposcopic assessment using digital colposcopic equipment. There are several major advantages to this technique, including the ability to store the image for future reference and an ability to undertake semi-quantitative assessments of the abnormal colposcopic findings. The image can be used for educational purposes (patients or those in training). As the image is stored digitally, it can be transmitted to other centres allowing telecolposcopy to be a feasible option especially when there are large distances to travel for colposcopic assessment or as an initial assessment for those women presenting with minor cervical cytological abnormalities.

DOCUMENTATION

This can either be performed using a specially designed colposcopy page, or data may be stored on a computer. Personal preferences will dictate this aspect, which is considered in more detail in Chapter 9.

TERMINOLOGY

One of the commonest methods of detailing the colposcopy findings is hand-drawn documentation. Diagrams can be added to printed outlines of the cervix, vagina or vulva. For the cervix, it is important to denote the limits of the native squamous epithelium and the transformation zone (TZ) and to show the new squamocolumnar junction (SCJ). The position of the anatomical external os should also be noted. Any areas of abnormality are carefully drawn and labelled (Figure 4.2).

PROBLEMS IN RUNNING A SERVICE

To run an effective cervical cancer prevention programme, we need as a minimum to have cytological screening, diagnostic colposcopy, facilities for histological

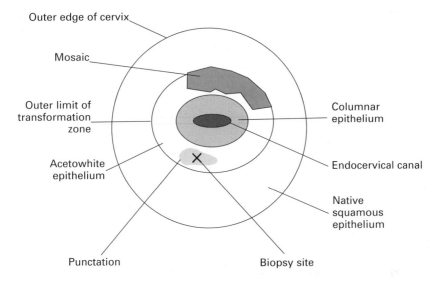

Figure 4.2 Diagrammatic representation of hand-drawn documentation commonly used to detail colposcopy findings.

diagnosis, treatment modalities and follow-up facilities. It is helpful if written guidelines are available in all clinics for the management of patients to cover most eventualities. Contacts between the cytologist, colposcopist and histopathologist are essential, and an audit programme of the service should be on-going. There should be good communication with the primary healthcare team (general practitioners), and with the patients themselves. Literature should be available for distribution to the patients, which explains the cervical cancer prevention programme and what will happen to them in the colposcopy clinic. This should be written in plain English and be easily understood.

The clinic layout should be both friendly and efficient. The overall set-up will be dependent upon the workload of the department, and may vary from a colposcopy room used intermittently to a dedicated facility with colposcopy services available most days.

TRAINING IN COLPOSCOPY

The standard of colposcopy practised in the UK varies from the excellent to the inadequate, and this situation is probably similar in most other countries. Other branches of medicine (e.g. ultrasound, psychosexual medicine and family planning) have recognized a similar problem and now offer a diploma or certificate of competence. It is important that women who attend for advice because of an abnormal smear are reassured that they are indeed being seen and advised by a colposcopist who is competent. Similarly, purchasers of colposcopy services need the reassurance that those services are being provided by competent colposcopists.

A system of accreditation in colposcopy will allow national organizations to recommend to purchasers that colposcopy clinics should only be supervised by those who have adequate accreditation, or even a diploma of colposcopy. Hospitals would have to ensure that adequately trained staff were employed to provide the colposcopy service. Similarly, in clinics staffed by non-specialists, colposcopists need some proof that they are indeed competent to provide the service. Chapter 18 deals with training and accreditation in more detail.

At the end of a training programme a trainee must:

- Be aware of the principles of cervical cytology, histopathology, pathophysiology and basic colposcopy.
- Be able to differentiate low-grade lesions, high-grade lesions and invasive disease of the lower genital tract.
- Be able to decide appropriate management and be thoroughly familiar with all surgical methods of treatment of pre-malignant and benign disease of the lower genital tract.
- Be able to counsel the woman with abnormal cytology or with a macroscopically abnormal cervix.

To achieve this, it is suggested that a training programme should consist of:

- Attendance at a basic colposcopy course.
- Performance of 50 colposcopic assessments on women presenting with abnormal cytology or suspicious lesions in the lower genital tract (direct supervision by a preceptor).
- Performance of 100 colposcopic examinations without direct supervision, each case subsequently being checked with the trainee by the preceptor.
- The trainee should be deemed competent by the preceptor to advise the woman of treatment options and to perform outpatient treatment, having previously performed this under supervision and to the satisfaction of the trainer.
- The trainee must be familiar with documentation and audit.
- In the future, no untrained personnel should be allowed to practise without: (i) having been properly trained; and (ii) having a certification of training in colposcopy.

LEARNING POINTS

- Colposcopy is a technique based upon magnification and illumination of the cervix.
- Magnification is usually between 6- and 40-fold.
- The patient should be warm, relaxed and informed.
- All basic instruments should be readily available before commencing a colposcopic examination.
- Sequential usage of saline, acetic acid and Lugol's iodine is recommended.
- The colposcopy findings need to be accurately documented using standard terminology.
- Training is vital prior to undertaking unsupervised colposcopy.

MCQs

For answers to Questions, see Appendix C.

10. **With regard to the history of colposcopy:**
    a. Colposcopy was introduced by Hans Hinselmann.
    b. Colposcopy is complementary to cervical cytology.
    c. Commonly used magnifications are up to 200-fold.
    d. The focal length varies between 200 and 300 mm.
    e. The blue filter has been an important development in the field of colposcopy.

11. **With regard to equipment in the colposcopy clinic:**
    a. The smallest speculum available should be used.
    b. Iris hooks can be useful for manipulation.
    c. Lugol's iodine is a useful stain to detect pre-invasive disease.
    d. An endocervical speculum is useful for examining the lower endocervical canal.
    e. Biopsies should be taken randomly from the cervical transformation zone.

12. **During a colposcopic examination:**
    a. The cervix should be partially exposed.
    b. Assessment of the angioarchitecture is important.
    c. Normal squamous epithelium fails to stain with acetic acid.
    d. Areas of metaplasia are abnormal, and should be excised.
    e. Acetowhite lesions extending onto the vagina may be encountered in some instances.

chapter 5

NORMAL COLPOSCOPIC APPEARANCES

J. Murphy

INTRODUCTION

In earlier chapters of this text the anatomy of the cervix was presented in detail. In addition, the various cervical epithelia, their appearance and their relationship to the development of cervical cancer have been outlined. The importance of colposcopy in the understanding of the pathophysiology of the cervix was also highlighted, as was a description on colposcopic technique.

Colposcopy, with its unique ability to examine *in situ* the epithelia of the cervix, has allowed the clinician to correlate the appearances of the cervix under direct vision with the histology of these tissues. Colposcopy has been the most significant advance in the management of women with abnormal cervical cytology, and the colposcopic appearances of abnormal cervical epithelia have allowed the clinician to direct the intelligent, and in most cases conservative, treatment of women with cervical intraepithelial neoplasia (CIN). The colposcopic appearances of the abnormal cervix are fascinating, and will be discussed in detail in subsequent chapters.

In common with all aspects of medicine, when considering the cervix, a thorough knowledge of the normal is an essential prerequisite for the study of the abnormal. This chapter examines the colposcopic appearances of normal cervical epithelia: squamous, columnar and metaplastic. The appearances of the normal subepithelial cervical vasculature will also be presented. A knowledge of the appearances of the three types of normal epithelia and the relationship between them is of first importance in understanding the origins of cervical cancer.

EPITHELIAL TYPES

The cervix has two fundamental types of epithelium: columnar and squamous, both of which are laid down *in utero* and meet each other in an abrupt fashion

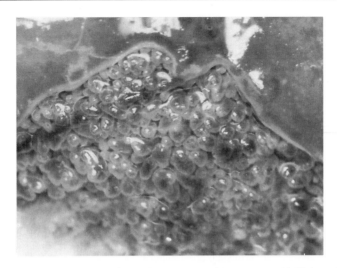

Figure 5.1 Normal columnar epithelium, showing normal squamous epithelium and the squamo-columnar junction. (Source: reproduced with permission from Malcolm Anderson, Joe Jordan, Anne Morse and Frank Sharp, *Integrated Colposcopy*, 2nd edition published in 1996 by Chapman & Hall, London.

at the original squamocolumnar junction (OSCJ) (Figure 5.1). In ideal, though somewhat theoretical, circumstances the OSCJ is situated at the external os, but depending on the size, shape and configuration of the external os, various proportions of the endocervical canal may be visible.

The position of the OSCJ is variable. It may be completely within the endo-cervical canal and consequently invisible to the unaided eye (or even to the colpo-scopist), or it may encroach for a variable degree on to the ectocervix being, in this situation, often described as an ectopy. Using the unaided eye, columnar epithelium appears red; this is because the epithelium is very thin and the blood vessels of each columnar villus give a characteristic red colour.

COLUMNAR EPITHELIUM

At colposcopy, normal epithelium is relatively easy to recognize because of its villus or 'grape-like' appearance. Before the application of acetic acid, and at high colpo-scopic magnification, it can be observed that each villus has a central blood vessel. The blood in the capillaries passes through the single layer of cells and gives the characteristic appearance. Contact bleeding is consequently common, and the epithelial surface can be easily damaged. When acetic acid is applied, the villi often appear white and are in general more distinct. At very high magnification with the

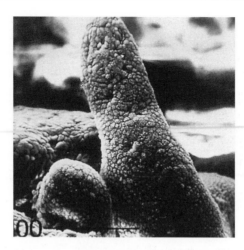

Figure 5.2 Scanning electron micrograph of a columnar epithelial villus. Each villus is covered by columnar cells. (Source: reproduced with permission from Malcolm Anderson, Joe Jordan, Anne Morse and Frank Sharp, *Integrated Colposcopy*, 2nd edition published in 1996 by Chapman & Hall, London.

scanning or surface electron microscope, each columnar villus is covered by a myriad of columnar cells each of which in turn is covered by microvilli (Figure 5.2).

SQUAMOUS EPITHELIUM

With colposcopy, two types of squamous epithelium may be recognized: original squamous epithelium, and transformed or metaplastic squamous epithelium. The original squamous epithelium, which is formed during fetal development, covers a variable part of the ectocervix and is similar to the squamous epithelium of the vagina except that stromal papillae are less frequent, or even absent. At colposcopy, using ordinary light, it appears smooth, pale and pink in colour and has little apparent vascular pattern. However, if a green filter is interposed (the technique of Kraatz) in most cases the underlying capillary network becomes apparent (Figure 5.3).

This network takes the form of tiny, hairpin-like capillaries that are densely arranged, particularly around the external os. When examined at very high magnification with the scanning electron microscope, squamous epithelium is composed of large flat cells with well-developed nuclei arranged in a pavement-like pattern. The surface of these cells is composed of microridges, which interdigitate with those of cells in the lower layers, thus giving this type of epithelium its characteristic strength.

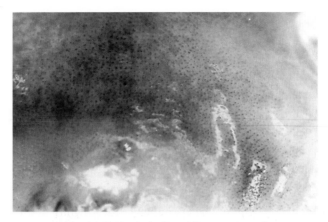

Figure 5.3 Fine hairpin capillaries. The intercapillary difference varies between 50 and 200 (µm). (Source: reproduced with permission from Malcolm Anderson, Joe Jordan, Anne Morse and Frank Sharp, *Integrated Colposcopy*, 2nd edition published in 1996 by Chapman & Hall, London.

METAPLASTIC SQUAMOUS EPITHELIA

To begin to understand the origins of cervical cancer and to use colposcopy intelligently, a knowledge of squamous metaplasia is essential. This process has already been extensively discussed in previous chapters. It has been accepted, now for some decades, that columnar epithelium exposed to the vaginal environment tends to change into squamous epithelium by the process of squamous metaplasia. The term 'transformation zone' (TZ) is used by the colposcopist to describe that part of the cervix which at one stage in its life had been covered by columnar epithelium, but which subsequently changed to squamous epithelium by the process of metaplasia.

Therefore the TZ is an area of variable width and configuration lying between the columnar epithelium and the original squamous epithelium. This area contains areas of columnar epithelium and metaplastic squamous epithelium of various stages of maturity. It also contains cervical crypt openings, and at times Nabothian cysts. These cysts occur when a crypt opening becomes covered with metaplastic squamous epithelium and the mucus produced is unable to escape. In the pre-menopausal woman the TZ is usually wholly visible, whereas in the post-menopausal woman, consequent on cervical involution, it can be found in part or totally in the endocervical canal.

The distal limit of the TZ is easily defined, usually by a thin line separating the two squamous epithelia of different origin: the native and the metaplastic. This line also represents the position of the OSCJ.

RECOGNITION OF MATURE METAPLASIA

Mature metaplastic squamous epithelium can be difficult to distinguish from original squamous epithelium on superficial inspection. However, the presence of crypt openings and branching vessels (to be discussed later) are usually characteristic. Difficulty in interpretation can also arise from the coexistence of less mature metaplastic epithelium.

IMMATURE METAPLASIA

The early phases of the transformation from columnar to squamous epithelium can be difficult to recognize. The epithelium is acetowhite and can at times be confused with abnormal epithelium. Coppleson and Reid from Sydney, who did so much to make the whole entity of squamous metaplasia understandable, described three colposcopically recognizable stages of squamous metaplasia:

1. The columnar villi lose their translucency and each villus assumes a 'ground-glass' appearance.
2. The grape-like configuration disappears as successive villi are fused and the spaces between them are filled in.
3. The villus configuration is lost because of the fusion, and the end result is normal squamous epithelium (Figure 5.4).

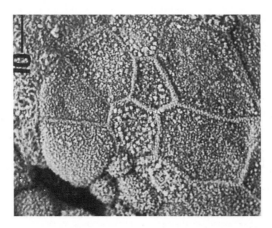

Figure 5.4 Metaplasia, Stage III. Scanning electron micrograph showing flat, almost mature squamous cells.(Source: reproduced with permission from Malcolm Anderson, Joe Jordan, Anne Morse and Frank Sharp, *Integrated Colposcopy*, 2nd edition published in 1996 by Chapman & Hall, London.

This metaplastic process is patchy however, and does not occur evenly and take place at the same time.

THE VASCULATURE OF THE NORMAL CERVIX

As a knowledge of the vascular pattern seen in epithelial abnormalities of the cervix is so important for their proper interpretation, it stands to reason that the appearances of the vessels in the normal cervix is also of significant importance. The part of the cervix covered with columnar epithelium is supplied by branches from the ascending branch of the uterine artery, while that part of the cervix covered by original squamous epithelium is supplied by branches from the cervicovaginal part of the uterine artery and by the vaginal artery. A well-developed network of vessels is then formed and the terminal aspects of these vessels can often be seen at colposcopy.

If squamous epithelium is examined in detail and with care, four types of capillaries may be identified. These were first described in detail by two Scandinavian colposcopists, Koller and Kolstad.

1. **Hairpin capillaries**: these terminal capillaries are formed by one ascending and one descending branch of fine calibre, forming a small loop. Usually only the tip of the loop is visible and the hairpin-like capillaries are recognized as regular and densely arranged small dots (see Figure 5.3).
2. **Network capillaries**: these are described when the terminal capillaries of the squamous epithelium form a dense, somewhat irregular meshwork of very fine vessels.
3. **Double capillaries**: this is the term applied to hairpin capillaries that show two or more crests at the top of the loop. They are characteristically found when there is inflammation of the cervical epithelium, particularly with *Trichomonas vaginalis*.
4. **Branching vessels**: these are larger terminal vessels showing irregular branching patterns (Figure 5.5). As they decrease in calibre, they terminate in a fine-mesh capillary network. They are characteristically seen in the TZ and are often prominent in the walls of retention Nabothian cysts. To the uninitiated, they might be confused with vascular patterns of invasive cancer, but with experience they can be easily distinguished.

CONCLUSION

It is axiomatic that a thorough knowledge of the normal is essential for understanding the abnormal. In company with other chapters in this text on normal

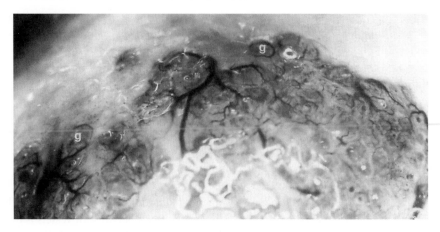

Figure 5.5 Branching vessels seen in a normal transformation zone. Some are arranged round a gland opening (g). (Source: reproduced with permission from Malcolm Anderson, Joe Jordan, Anne Morse and Frank Sharp, *Integrated Colposcopy*, 2nd edition published in 1996 by Chapman & Hall, London.

appearances and function, stress must be continually placed on the understanding and recognition of the phenomenon of squamous metaplasia.

LEARNING POINTS

- Columnar and squamous epithelium are the two basic epithelia laid down *in utero* and join at the original squamocolumnar junction.
- Columnar epithelium is one cell thick, hence it is easily traumatized.
- Colposcopy can identify original squamous and metaplastic squamous epithelium.
- The colposcopic transformation zone (TZ) represents an area of epithelium that at one stage in its development was columnar epithelium.
- The TZ is variable in width and configuration, and contains columnar and squamous metaplastic epithelium of varying maturity.
- The presence of crypt openings and branching vessels are characteristic of mature squamous metaplastic epithelium.
- Three stages of metaplasia can be identified colposcopically.

MCQs

For answers to Questions, see Appendix C.

13. **Regarding metaplasia:**
    a. Immature metaplasia stains white following acetic acid.
    b. A high vaginal pH causes squamous epithelium to change to columnar.
    c. Columnar epithelium cannot be present within the transformation zone.
    d. Fusion of villi in columnar epithelium is an early metaplastic event.
    e. The metaplastic process is patchy, uneven and irregular in timing.

14. **Regarding colposcopy:**
    a. Colposcopy cannot differentiate between original squamous and metaplastic epithelium.
    b. Gland openings confirm that the epithelium is original squamous epithelium.
    c. The distal limit of the transformation zone is usually easy to define.
    d. Double capillaries usually indicate an inflammatory process.
    e. Lugol's iodine is useful to study the vascular patterns on the cervix.

chapter 6

INDICATIONS FOR REFERRAL FOR COLPOSCOPY

I.D. Duncan

BACKGROUND

Hinselmann introduced the colposcope in 1925 to allow stereoscopic examination of the illuminated cervix under magnification. His main intention was to detect early cervical cancer, but he recommended the routine use of the colposcope for every woman undergoing gynaecological examination. The use of the colposcope in this way spread from Germany to Spain and other parts of mainland Europe, and from there to South America. The English-speaking world, including the UK, does not use colposcopy for primary screening for cervical premalignancy. Cervical cytology is routinely used in this respect, and the colposcope is reserved for those women in whom a diagnosis of cervical intraepithelial neoplasia (CIN) is suspected. Neither cytology nor colposcopy is 100% sensitive or specific, and false-negative and false-positive results occur with both methods. They are, however, complementary and the accuracy of using them in combination is greater than using either method in isolation. It is easier and quicker, however, to gain expertise in taking a smear than in carrying out colposcopy, and the cytological impression – unlike the colposcopic one – does not require the physical presence of the woman herself. For socioeconomic reasons, if for no other, it is highly unlikely that primary screening with colposcopy will become established as routine practice in the UK. It is important, therefore, that the indications for colposcopy are clearly set out.

GUIDELINES FOR REFERRAL

In 1981, the Working Party set up by the Royal College of Obstetricians and Gynaecologists recommended that no woman should be treated for CIN without first undergoing colposcopy (Jordan *et al.*, 1981). This recommendation remains sacrosanct. Priority should be given to the detection of CIN3 over CIN1, since the risk of CIN3 progressing through microinvasion to frank invasive cancer of the cervix is greater than for CIN1, which is more likely to regress to normality than is CIN3. The correlation between cytology and histology is not 100%, but it does approach this figure at the extremes, i.e. a woman with a negative smear is unlikely to have CIN, whilst a woman with severe dyskaryosis is likely to have high-grade CIN. In 1992, guidelines were published for clinical practice and programme management for use in the NHS Cervical Screening Programme (Duncan, 1992). In the light of experience, these guidelines were revised in 1997 (Duncan, 1997). Currently, these guidelines contain the recommendation that women with a smear showing moderate or severe dyskaryosis should be referred immediately for colposcopy.

Low-grade cervical cytology does not necessarily correlate with low-grade histological abnormality. Various centres have demonstrated the existence of CIN2 or 3 on colposcopically directed biopsy in women whose worst cytological abnormality is mild dyskaryosis (Lyall and Duncan, 1995). This is not because of faulty technique in either taking, preparing or reading the smear, but appears to be due to the fact that the high-grade lesion present in a woman with only mild dyskaryosis is very much smaller than when severe dyskaryosis is seen on the smear (Jarmulowicz *et al.*, 1989). Thus, a high-grade lesion must have a critical surface area before it is sufficiently represented on the smear, and the inaccuracy of low-grade cytology is a constant phenomenon. The National Guidelines recognize this and recommend that women with a borderline or mildly dyskaryotic smear should have it repeated 6 months later. If she has two mildly dyskaryotic smears, then she should be referred for colposcopy. Further discretion is exercised for women with persisting borderline abnormalities, the guidelines recommending a referral after three such smears at 6-monthly intervals unless the cytopathologist specifies difficulty in distinguishing the borderline changes from high-grade dyskaryosis, in which case colposcopy may be indicated earlier. The pros and cons of cytological surveillance versus prompt referral for colposcopy are the subject of large multicentre studies currently being conducted both in the UK and overseas.

Colposcopy should be considered the first time a woman has a mildly dyskaryotic smear if this smear follows treatment for CIN, or if it is anticipated that the woman will not comply with smear follow-up.

OTHER REFERRAL SITUATIONS

Although the basis for colposcopic referral is abnormal cytology, there are other situations in which colposcopy may be useful. In some young women the degree of cervical eversion and the fragility of the exposed columnar epithelium is such that the cervix bleeds readily when a smear is taken. In this case the number of red blood cells may be sufficient to obscure the cervical cells, so that the smear is reported as unsatisfactory (see Chapter 2). If the smears are unsatisfactory on three occasions, the National Guidelines recommend referral to the colposcopist in order that the woman's cervix can be examined and pronounced normal, or not.

In the UK, cervical screening is predominantly carried out in primary care, and with increasing frequency by the practice nurse who is increasingly unlikely to encounter cervical cancer. Benign conditions, for example condylomata acuminata, can give rise to the suspicion of cancer, and even if the cytology is negative the exceptional case should be referred for colposcopic examination.

PRIMARY SCREENING COLPOSCOPY

Primary screening with colposcopy is sometimes used in genitourinary medicine clinics. In the UK the population attending these clinics tends to be younger women with a higher prevalence of human papillomavirus (HPV) infection and CIN (especially low-grade) than the general population as a whole. Concomitant sexually transmitted inflammatory conditions of the cervix such as infection with *Trichomonas vaginalis* or *Chlamydia trachomatis* may again render cytology less reliable and the addition of colposcopy a useful adjunct.

COLPOSCOPY OF OTHER STRUCTURES

Although primarily designed for examination of the cervix, the colposcope can be used to look at other structures such as the vulva or penis. The vascular pattern is less apparent in these structures since the skin is thicker than the cervical epithelium. Nuclear-rich tissues will still temporarily turn white after the application of acetic acid, although the process is slower than in the cervix. Vulvar intraepithelial neoplasia (VIN) and penile intraepithelial neoplasia (PIN) are much less common than CIN. VIN is usually symptomatic, the commonest symptom being pruritus or soreness. The lesions may be seen with the naked eye and are commonly multifocal; they may be red or brown, or white if there is increased keratinization present. Penile lesions may be unsuspected, but can be located on the shaft of the penis of the male partners of women with CIN, especially those with persistent or recurrent CIN. A hand lens as used by the dermatologist can be a simple substitute for the colposcope.

The carbon dioxide laser is still commonly used to treat these lesions, despite the fact that recurrence is likely; of course, the colposcope is usually an integral part of such a laser system.

CONCLUSION

Squamous cervical cancer is largely preventable. Well-established cytology programmes have been rewarded by a fall in incidence of the condition, but false-negative results still occur. In addition, large numbers of women with minor lesions – the vast majority of which are not pre-cancerous – are caught in the net and end up being investigated and often treated. Trials are under way checking the HPV status of women when the smear is taken. HPV 16 and 18 are the more common of the so-called high-risk oncogenic group, and are associated with high-grade intraepithelial neoplasia and cancer, while HPV 6 and 11 are characteristic of the low-risk group and predominate in low-grade lesions. Again, correlation between histology and HPV status is not 100%. A few low-grade lesions will contain high-risk virus, and a few high-grade lesions will contain low-risk virus. In the future it is possible that HPV status may be used to refine referral for colposcopy.

The National Guidelines also contain recommendations for the follow-up of women who have undergone treatment for CIN and in whom cytology is essential. Colposcopy has been shown to aid in the early detection of persistent lesions, and may be used at the 6-month follow-up visit. The National Guidelines recommend its use at this visit if excision has been employed to eradicate CIN and the margins are doubtful or if microinvasive cancer or high-grade cervical glandular intraepithelial neoplasia (CGIN) have been treated by excision of the transformation zone. If, however, that examination is negative it need not be repeated.

Women in the UK find colposcopy at best distasteful and at worst a frightening, humiliating procedure. Referral for colposcopy must, therefore, be a careful balance between the benefits likely to accrue to the woman and the psychological trauma of an unnecessary intrusive examination.

LEARNING POINTS

- Moderate and severe dyskaryosis are indications for referral for colposcopy.
- Any suspicious-looking cervical lesion is an indication for referral, regardless of the cytology report.
- Mild dyskaryosis and borderline changes should prompt a repeat smear 6 months after the index smear. If any abnormality persists, referral is

recommended. These guidelines are based upon a common consensus, and not on the evidence of clinical trials.

- Colposcopy is not generally regarded as a screening process.
- Between 20% and 40% of women who have low-grade smear reports (mild dyskaryosis and borderline nuclear abnormalities) will have CIN2 or CIN3 on biopsy. These lesions tend to be smaller than those presenting with high-grade cytological abnormalities.
- The colposcope is primarily designed for examination of the cervix. Examination of other areas of the female lower genital tract and the penis may be enhanced by its use.

MCQs

For answers to Questions, see Appendix C.

15. **The following are indications for colposcopy in the UK:**
    a. A single mildly dyskaryotic smear.
    b. A single moderately dyskaryotic smear.
    c. A single severely dyskaryotic smear.
    d. A cervical polyp.
    e. A routine follow-up visit 18 months after treatment for CIN3.

16. **Which of the following statements are true?**
    a. There is a high correlation between negative cytology and negative histology.
    b. There is a high correlation between low-grade cytology and low-grade histology.
    c. There is a high correlation between high-grade cytology and high-grade histology.
    d. HPV 16 is a high-risk oncogenic virus.
    e. HPV 6 is a high-risk oncogenic virus.

17. **Which of the following statements about colposcopy are true?**
    a. It was first developed in Germany.
    b. It is used as a screening tool in some genitourinary medicine clinics in the UK.
    c. It is usually performed at a magnification of ×40.
    d. It is only used to examine female anatomy.
    e. It is essential in the diagnosis of VIN.

chapter 7

COLPOSCOPY OF THE ATYPICAL TRANSFORMATION ZONE

J. Cordiner

INTRODUCTION

The transformation zone (TZ) is that area of the cervix whose limits define cervical intraepithelial neoplasia (CIN). A comprehensive understanding of the normal anatomy, the physiology and colposcopy is necessary to interpret abnormal findings. Unfortunately, there is no single feature capable of defining a distinct histological abnormality.

It is important that the cervix be viewed prior to the application of acetic acid, as many of the features suggestive of CIN are present when viewed microscopically, especially when accentuated by gently cleansing the area with saline and visualizing with a green filter *in situ*. However, the majority of colposcopy clinics in the UK will use the acetic acid technique in order to delineate the abnormal TZ.

THE ATYPICAL TZ

ACETOWHITE EPITHELIUM

This is a focal abnormal colposcopic appearance after the application of acetic acid (Plate 2). It is a transient phenomenon associated with increased nuclear density, and is the most commonly found of all abnormal features associated with the abnormal TZ. It is not diagnostic of CIN, however. Acetowhite epithelium may be found in association with human papillomavirus (HPV) infection, immature squamous metaplasia, congenital transformation zone and regenerating epithelium.

In general, the more intense the change, the more extreme the degree of histological abnormality. The ectocervical edge may be clear and well-defined or fuzzy, the latter often being associated with HPV infection.

VASCULAR PATTERN

The viewed pattern and calibre of the subepithelial capillaries frequently give a striking colposcopic appearance. There are three clearly identifiable types.

Mosaic

This is a focal abnormal colposcopic appearance in which the vascular patterns show fields of mosaic within the transformation zone (Plate 3). The capillaries appear parallel to the surface, giving the characteristic crazy-paving pattern. The calibre of the capillaries may vary, as may the surface area enclosed. The wider the calibre and the greater the surface area enclosed, the more likely a greater degree of abnormality.

Punctation

The stromal capillaries produce a stippled or punctate appearance within the epithelium (Plate 4). The degree of punctation may be fine with evenly spaced loop capillaries of narrow calibre with minimal intercapillary distance. In a more marked change, the course and calibre of the capillaries is altered, with coarse-calibre vessels often called (and resembling) 'corkscrews'. In general, the more severe the change the greater the degree of histological abnormality. In many inflammatory states the subepithelial capillaries open up and again produce a stippled effect.

This should not be confused with punctation associated with an abnormal transformation zone as the punctation in inflammatory change is diffuse and extends on to the original squamous epithelium in the vagina and fornices.

Atypical vessels

These vessels are frequently arranged in a haphazard way (Plate 5). New vessels are formed and often demonstrate gross variation in calibre and branching. At the extreme, the appearances of atypical vessels are suggestive that early invasion of the stroma may have taken place. The vessels themselves are different from vascular patterns seen in the normal transformation zone. Fine terminal branching is uncommon with atypical vessels.

If acetic acid is used, the vascular appearance of the TZ may be obliterated by dense acetowhite epithelium. The pattern may not be obvious until the effect of the acetic acid wears off.

GRADING OF COLPOSCOPIC FINDINGS

There is no one feature of the abnormal transformation zone which is diagnostic. Consequently, it has been customary to grade the findings:

- Grade I: the epithelium is flat and white with fine-calibre, regular blood vessels and a small intercapillary distance.
- Grade II: the epithelium remains flat, but is whiter after the application of acetic acid. The vessels are usually regular but perhaps of a larger diameter, with increased intercapillary distance.
- Grade III: the epithelium is intensely acetowhite; the blood vessels are dilated and irregular with frequently a variable intercapillary distance. There may also be atypical vessels present. The surface in early invasive cancer may be uneven, papillary or exophytic. The variations of the surface contour, and the vessels are often coincident but one may exist without the other. The appearance of atypical vessels and a grossly irregular surface contour is highly suggestive of invasive carcinoma.

LEUKOPLAKIA

This is a focal appearance in which there is hyperkeratosis or parakeratosis. It appears on colposcopy as an elevated, roughened, white area prior to the application of acetic acid. Some of the keratin may be washed away using a saline-soaked swab, thereby leaving a glistening whitened appearance. It may be patchy, or it may cover large areas of the cervix and extend outside the TZ on to the vagina. Its significance is that it may obscure visualization of the surface and vascular architecture of the TZ. Biopsy is required.

VAGINAL EXTENSION OF CIN

In the majority of cases encountered in women of reproductive years, it will be possible to visualize the whole transformation zone on the cervix. In a small number of cases (about 5%) there may be vaginal extension of the TZ on to the vaginal vault. This may occur for two reasons:

1. **Vaginal extension of intraepithelial disease:** here, there has been genuine metaplastic/dysplastic change taking place on the extended TZ. The

appearances colposcopically will be similar to those on the cervix, with acetowhite epithelium and altered angioarchitecture. The limits are often well-defined after application of Lugol's iodine, as the area does not take up the iodine stain.

2. **Congenital transformation zone**: this concept is often confusing to both experienced and inexperienced colposcopists. Under normal circumstances, columnar epithelium undergoing the physiological change of metaplasia reaches full maturation, the resulting squamous epithelium being indistinguishable from normal. In a small but often confusing number of patients, the metaplastic change results in an acetowhite epithelium which is non-glycogenated. The majority of this change is on the cervix, but it may extend on to the vaginal vault; this is termed the congenital TZ. On visualization of this after the application of acetic acid, it is often slow to become white and slow to return to normal. There is often an extremely fine mosaic of thin-calibre vessels on its surface and the epithelium is poorly or non-glycogenated. The appearances are often confusing, and frequently biopsy is required to confirm the classic histological features of the congenital TZ. Its potential for malignancy is low and treatment is not required.

ENDOCERVICAL EXTENSION OF THE TZ

While in cases of CIN the ectocervical limits of a lesion are often clear and well demarcated, the endocervical limits are frequently less well defined. In many women in late reproductive life or who may be post-menopausal, the TZ will extend to beyond the visual limits of the colposcope. An endocervical speculum may be helpful to define the upper limit, but as the incident light from the colposcope is not at right-angles to the lesion, the appearances can occasionally be confusing. Excision biopsy should be undertaken should there be any doubt about the upper limit of the TZ.

HPV APPEARANCES AND COLPOSCOPY

There is increasing evidence of the strong association between HPV and the development of cervical pre-cancer and cancer. Colposcopic evidence of HPV infection may vary from clearly defined exophytic warts through non-condylomatous warts, and indeed to virtually normal colposcopic appearances.

CONDYLOMA ACUMINATA

The classical lesions of wart virus infection may be visible to the naked eye. They have multiple papillary projections, each with its own looped capillary. An important feature is that such lesions are not confined to the TZ but also extend out on to the vagina and to the lower genital tract. On colposcopy, each individual wart has a frond-like surface and central capillary that is often better visualized before the application of acetic acid. With the application of acetic acid there is intense blanching of the surface that frequently persists for some time. Occasionally, the surface of the wart has an appearance likened to the human brain (encephaloid appearance) in which the surface is heaped up and has a whorled appearance. As such lesions are frequently associated with CIN, biopsy is often required.

FLAT WARTS (NON-CONDYLOMATOUS WART VIRUS INFECTION)

Documentation of the classical appearance of subclinical papillomavirus infections is difficult as the appearances are often subtle and indistinct. The surface of the epithelium is often shiny and off-white, whilst the margins of the lesion are often irregular and pointed and have a feathery appearance. There may indeed be satellite lesions outside the TZ. There may be fine punctation with a fine mosaic pattern of the underlying vessels. Several authors have attempted to score appearances to simplify the classification, but although these may be helpful in the training of the colposcopist, biopsy of the lesion is often the only way to determine whether underlying CIN is present.

UNSATISFACTORY COLPOSCOPY

It is the function of colposcopy and the colposcopist to be able to define the outer and inner limits of the TZ, to make an interpretation of these findings, and to enable appropriate biopsy and treatment to be undertaken. Colposcopy is deemed to be unsatisfactory when it is not possible to do this. It may be a simple fact that visualization of the cervix is poor or that the TZ extends into the endocervical canal and outside the visual range. In certain circumstances, coexisting lesions may cause some confusion.

INFLAMMATORY CHANGES

A wide range of causes exist for this. Common organisms such as *Candida albicans*, *Trichomonas vaginalis* and *Neisseria gonorrhoeae* may produce a severe vascular response. On colposcopy, the appearances are compatible with hyper-aemia of the vascular capillary bed. The terminal capillaries become dilated and often looped in an accentuated normal response. This produces an intense punc-tation but, in contradistinction to the atypical TZ, the vessels are close together and will usually extend on to the vaginal epithelium.

ATROPHIC EPITHELIUM

Colposcopy of oestrogen-deficient epithelium is often confusing. The epithelium becomes pale, white and thin, and the full subepithelial network of capillaries is often visualized through the thinned epithelium. Subepithelial haemorrhage is common.

TRUE EROSION

This is an area of denuded epithelium, usually caused by trauma. On colposcopy, the exposed area is red, as the terminal vessels are visualized. The epithelium is lifted off the crater base and can be easily identified.

SUMMARY

It is important that the colposcopist detects the abnormal colposcopic appearances of pre-malignant and early malignant disease. As has been emphasized, no one appearance is classical, and appearances can often be confusing. Biopsy of any areas of doubt is the only method to determine whether treatment is required or not.

LEARNING POINTS

- No one colposcopic feature is diagnostic of cervical intraepithelial neoplasia (CIN).
- The vascular pattern of the subendothelial capillary network should be first assessed after the application of normal saline and using a green filter.
- In general, the coarser the vascular pattern and more intense the whiteness after the application of acetic acid, the worse the degree of CIN.
- Human papillomavirus (HPV) and immature metaplasia may also result in acetowhite changes.
- Atypical vessels and an irregular surface contour are suggestive of underlying invasion.
- Leukoplakia can mask underlying CIN.

- Acetowhite epithelium extending on to the vagina may represent either true dysplastic extension (VaIN) or a congenital transformation zone (TZ).
- The colposcopic features of HPV infection are subtle, and can be confused with mild dysplastic change. Extension of atypicality beyond the TZ is, however, suggestive of HPV.
- Inflammatory processes can cause marked changes in the subepithelial capillary network that also extend beyond the TZ.

CLINICAL CASE SCENARIO 1

A 22-year-old para 0+0 is referred for colposcopy with a smear showing mild dyskaryosis on two occasions. On colposcopic examination, an initial assessment reveals no abnormality.

Acetic acid (5%) is applied to reveal the following:

- The whole TZ is seen.
- The anterior lip of the cervix reveals faint acetowhite epithelium grade I, with a faint edge to the ectocervical margin of the TZ.
- There is a mosaic pattern of the vessels.
- The posterior lip reveals the acetowhite change to be more dense (grade II), with clear evidence of mosaic pattern of blood vessels.
- There are no abnormal vessels.

Questions

1. What do the colposcopic findings suggest?
2. Is this compatible with the smear report?
3. What is the minimum number of biopsies that should be taken?
4. Does the appearance suggest an invasive lesion?
5. What form of treatments may be appropriate when biopsy results are available?

MCQs

For answers to Questions, see Appendix C.

18. **Acetowhite change may be seen in the following conditions:**
    a. CIN.
    b. Wart virus infection.

    c. Metaplasia.

    d. Invasive squamous carcinoma.

    e. Congenital transformation zone.

19. **If atypical blood vessels are seen on colposcopy:**

    a. A punch biopsy is required to rule out invasion.

    b. The lesion may be treated with cold coagulation.

    c. This gives rise to suspicion of an invasive lesion.

    d. They may be ignored if the smear shows mild dyskaryosis.

    e. They are commonly seen on the surface of nabothian follicles.

20. **CIN:**

    a. Can always be diagnosed on colposcopy.

    b. Can be diagnosed with the naked eye.

    c. Is never found in association with condyloma accuminata of the cervix.

    d. Can be diagnosed with a colposcope without use of acetic acid.

    e. Is excluded if the smear is normal.

chapter 8

ABNORMAL COLPOSCOPY (EARLY INVASION, GLANDULAR LESIONS)

C.W.E. Redman

INTRODUCTION

This chapter focuses on the colposcopic assessment of early invasive and glandular cervical lesions. The term 'glandular lesions' can embrace a histopathogical spectrum of endocervical abnormality from low-grade cervical glandular intraepithelial neoplasia (LGCGIN), via the more severe high-grade cervical glandular intraepithelial neoplasia (HGCGIN) to frank invasive adenocarcinoma. In this chapter, only HGCGIN and adenocarcinoma will be considered. Early invasion is synonymous with the term pre-clinical cancer, i.e. FIGO stages Ia_1 to Ia_2. Histopathological aspects and management are described elsewhere.

Colposcopy is necessary for optimal management of women with abnormal cervical cytology or suspicious clinical features, but the actual colposcopic assessment *per se* provides only part of the necessary information. Other important clinical features include the history, examination findings and other investigations. This chapter aims to describe the detection and assessment of early invasive and glandular lesion more fully than simply to detail what might be seen looking down a colposcope. There are no colposcopic features diagnostic of a glandular lesion. The colposcope merely serves to increase suspicion of such a lesion. Diagnosis is histological.

THE IMPORTANCE OF EARLY INVASIVE AND GLANDULAR LESIONS

Histopathologically, these lesions occupy a grey area between pre-invasive and frankly invasive cancer, and this is reflected in attitudes and recommendations about treatment. Appropriate treatment depends on accurate diagnosis, and it is now clear that prior to the advent of loop diathermy excision these lesions were significantly underdiagnosed and undertreated, even by expert colposcopists. The clinical challenge posed by these lesions has diminished with the increasing use of loop diathermy.

INDEX OF SUSPICION

Such severe lesions are at one end of the spectrum of disease that is seen in a colposcopy clinic, and are uncommon. There is therefore a danger that these cases can easily be overlooked against a background of accompanying minor pathology. Such lesions are too uncommon to be targeted specifically by the screening programme that aims at detecting and treating high-grade disease, principally CIN3. There are, however, certain features other than cytology that should alert the clinician to the possibility of invasive disease.

SYMPTOMS

Post-coital, inter-menstrual and of course post-menopausal bleeding are all symptoms that have a sinister significance until proven otherwise. In the UK, national guidelines recommend that such cases should be referred to a gynaecologist, and if the suspicion of cancer is high the patient should be referred to the gynaecological cancer team. When cervical cancer is suspected, urgent colposcopy is required. A cervical smear should not be taken in these circumstances. In the case of genuine post-coital bleeding there is an argument for assessment to include routinely cervical loop diathermy excision.

PAST HISTORY

A previous history of treatment for a high-grade cervical lesion, particularly if the lesion was incompletely excised or if the treatment was ablative, should lower the threshold of suspicion. In any event the proven limitations of colposcopy following treatment make histological assessment important should problems arise.

EXAMINATION FINDINGS

In addition to the clinical appearance of the cervix, bimanual examination may raise the possibility of frank invasion because the cervix feels both hard and irregular or abnormal in shape or size. However, early invasive lesions will be subclinical.

COLPOSCOPIC FEATURES SUGGESTING INVASION

Invasive lesions may be clinically apparent, presenting with ulceration or obvious topographical hypertrophy. However, not all lesions will be clinically apparent when a patient is first seen. Classically a number of colposcopic features are considered to be suggestive of invasion. These features simply represent one end of a spectrum of the colposcopic grading of atypical lesions, and may not all be evident in any given case. Before the application of acetic acid, invasion may be obvious from the bizarre appearance of the cervix, if the surface is grossly distorted or ulcerated, or from the presence of abnormal vessels. By and large, the application of acetic acid accentuates the features that indicate microinvasive disease (Plates 6 and 7).

ABNORMAL VESSELS

Markedly atypical and prominent vessels are said to be the hallmark, and can have a number of appearances:

- Coarse irregular vessels with a variety of forms (e.g. 'corkscrew' and 'comma') (Plates 8 and 9).
- Coarse punctation.
- 'Atypical vessels' – those seen with irregular calibre and usually irregular branching with a wide intercapillary distance.
- These features are often very prominent if the lesion is hypertrophic. When there is ulceration they are less obvious.

IRREGULAR SURFACE

The presence of an uneven or raised surface must suggest the possibility of invasion. Invasive cancer is characterized by an irregular and exophytic growth pattern.

LARGE, COMPLEX LESION

There is a positive correlation between lesion size and the histological severity. The larger the lesion, the more likely it is to be high-grade. Complex patterns represent a combination of acetowhite, mosaic and punctation.

SEVERE CHANGES WITH CANAL INVOLVEMENT

Any of these features would suggest that an adequate biopsy, such as loop diathermy excision or formal knife cone biopsy is indicated.

PROBLEMS IN THE RECOGNITION OF EARLY INVASION

Colposcopy may suggest early invasion when it is not there (false positive) or, more worryingly, miss it when it is there (false negative). Overall, colposcopy has not been shown to be particularly accurate, especially in the context of microinvasive disease. It should be regarded as a technique for guiding biopsy and treatment by indicating the likely underlying histological diagnosis in conjunction with other data items, such as cytology, smoking and past history.

False positives are not a major problem. They may result in some unnecessary intervention, but most of these lesions will nonetheless be high-grade CIN if not invasive lesions and therefore would require treatment in any event. When invasion is suspected, histological confirmation prior to more extensive therapy is mandatory and at this stage the error will be detected. Such errors should be unusual, although the number will depend on the individual's threshold for making such decisions. False positives are more likely in pregnancy, as the vascular pattern tends to be exaggerated.

False negatives are, on the other hand, an important problem because early invasive lesions will either not be treated appropriately or even not treated at all. The advent of loop diathermy excision has resulted in an increase in the incidence of early invasion, even in centres of excellence, which means that early invasive lesions were previously missed and inappropriately managed.

A number of factors make false negatives more common:

- **Previous treatment:** the scarring and deformation of the cervical transformation zone (TZ) resulting from previous treatment, particularly if ablative, makes colposcopy unreliable.
- **Endocervical lesions:** colposcopy cannot assess any lesion that is hidden from view, for instance when the squamocolumnar junction (SCJ) is within the endocervical canal.
- **Leukoplakia:** this is not itself indicative of malignancy, but as it may mask an underlying lesion it should be biopsied.

- **Pregnancy**: there is a natural tendency to avoid any intervention in pregnancy, and therefore a reluctance to perform colposcopy. Colposcopy can be more technically demanding and its findings difficult to interpret.

CAN GLANDULAR LESIONS BE RECOGNIZED?

Frankly invasive adenocarcinoma or adenosquamous carcinoma of the cervix will have similar appearances to squamous lesions. However, there are major limitations in the colposcopic assessment of suspected glandular lesions as severe pre-invasive glandular lesions such as HGCGIN have no typical colposcopic appearance. The only clue may be increased fragility or coexistent CIN.

Frankly invasive glandular lesions will present in a similar manner to the more common squamous cancers. HGCGIN presents either as an abnormal glandular smear or is found coincidentally in the course of the management of squamous dyskaryosis. Abnormal glandular smears have a variety of forms ranging from 'endometrial' cells being found in cervical smears in inappropriate phases of the menstrual cycle to more marked glandular dyskaryosis through to the positive detection of adenocarcinoma cells. The possibility of HGCGIN or worse has to be considered throughout the spectrum of these cytological reports, although most 'glandular' smears are only mild and not associated with any significant pathology.

COLPOSCOPIC ASSESSMENT WHEN SMEARS HAVE MILD GLANDULAR ABNORMALITIES

There is an argument that loop diathermy is indicated in the assessment of all women having smears showing a glandular abnormality, as this is the only way satisfactorily to assess the endocervical canal. This would be an overreaction, as most mildly glandular smears need not reflect underlying dysplasia. Currently assessment includes:

- Consideration of whether there may be endometrial pathology and performing an endometrial sample if indicated.
- Performing an endocervical cytobrush examination – if this provides further evidence of cytological atypia then loop diathermy excision should be performed.

ASSESSMENT WHEN INVASION OR SEVERE GLANDULAR LESIONS ARE SUSPECTED COLPOSCOPICALLY

HISTOLOGICAL CONFIRMATION

In these circumstances histological confirmation is mandatory. The biopsy must be sufficient to allow adequate pathological assessment. Histology can be inadequate in two ways. First, not enough material may be provided, and in this respect a punch biopsy is totally inadequate. Few colposcopists would knowingly use a punch biopsy to confirm a colposcopic diagnosis of microinvasion, but early invasive lesions are often not suspected colposcopically. It follows that punch biopsies are of dubious value. Second, the diagnosis of microinvasion or HGCGIN can only be safely made when the entire lesion has been removed, which may be better assessed after a knife cone biopsy as opposed to a loop diathermy, as the margins of excision are clearer.

If frank invasion may be suspected, it is pointless performing a large cone biopsy with its attendant dangers to confirm a diagnosis that is clinically obvious. In this circumstance a piece of cervix can be removed either digitally or using a loop.

In the UK, national guidelines recommend that if early invasion is suspected, a designated pathologist should examine the biopsy specimen. The pathologist should have a special interest in malignant gynaecological disease. Any specimens thought to show cancer should also be sent to a specialist pathologist at a cancer centre to check the findings.

Whenever an early invasive lesion is suspected, a bimanual pelvic examination should be performed to exclude the possibility of local extension. Other investigations such as chest X-ray and intravenous urogram can be deferred until histology is to hand.

REFERRAL TO THE GYNAECOLOGICAL CANCER TEAM

In the UK, women with cervical squamous cell carcinoma (FIGO stage Ia$_2$ or greater) or an adenocarcinoma should be referred to the specialist gynaecological oncology team at a cancer centre.

LEARNING POINTS

- Markedly abnormal vessels are highly suggestive of early invasive disease.
- Despite there being well-described colposcopic features, microinvasive lesions are frequently underdiagnosed.

- If microinvasion is suspected, adequate histological confirmation is mandatory.
- Glandular lesions have no reliable colposcopic features.

CLINICAL CASE SCENARIO 2

A 46-year-old patient presented with a 'positive' glandular smear, suggestive of endocervical carcinoma. She was asymptomatic and had regular, normal periods. Her previous cervical smears had been normal. She was nulliparous and a non-smoker. She needed no contraception but had been on the oral contraceptive 'pill' in the past. Colposcopy was unremarkable; the examination was satisfactory, the squamocolumnar junction was seen, and no abnormality was noted. Bimanual examination was normal. After discussion, an endometrial sample and an extended loop diathermy cone was performed. Histology was requested urgently and the specimen was found to contain HGCGIN. There was no evidence of invasive cancer, but it was not possible to be sure that the HGCGIN had been completely excised. The endometrial sample was normal. The options were discussed, which ranged from cytological follow-up to hysterectomy. Further excision was advised and the patient opted for knife conization. This specimen contained no residual disease and arrangements were made for follow-up in the colpscopy clinic in 6 months' time.

Questions

1. How urgently should patients with smears such as this be seen? What investigations are appropriate? How do women with CGIN normally present?
2. What factors have been implicated in the aetiology of CGIN?
3. What is the most appropriate biopsy for suspected CGIN, and why?
4. Is bimanual examination always necessary in women referred with such smears? If so why does this differ from the norm?
5. What is the rationale for the types of acceptable management?

MCQs

For answers to Questions, see Appendix C.

21. **Regarding HGCGIN:**
    a. Patients usually present with abnormal bleeding.
    b. It has well-defined colposcopic features.

   c. Cone biopsy is only useful as a diagnostic procedure.
   d. Frequently presents with coexistent squamous lesions.
   e. Pregnancy changes may mask the usual colposcopic features.

22. **The following statements are true:**
   a. When glandular lesions are suspected, excisional biopsy must be performed.
   b. When frank invasion is apparent, diagnostic cone biopsy is mandatory.
   c. Coarse punctation is a typical feature of HGCGIN.
   d. Early invasive lesions are likely to have wide intercapillary distances.
   e. Acetic acid application can mask abnormal vascular patterns.

23. **Regarding early invasive lesions:**
   a. Cervical cytology is highly predictive.
   b. Knife cone is best avoided.
   c. Patients with Stage Ia_2 disease should be referred to a cancer centre for further management.
   d. Local treatment, using ablation, is acceptable.

chapter 9

RECORDING THE INFORMATION

D.M. Luesley

INTRODUCTION

Colposcopic assessments, just like any other form of medical assessment, require documentation. This is important for clinical use (future visits), audit and research. Established clinics have now developed standard formats for note-taking and image-recording, and these usually take the form of a structured or semistructured form for recording important aspects of the history and relevant clinical findings. It must be stressed that colposcopy clinics are specialized clinics for the assessment and management of women with abnormal cervical smears or clinically suspicious cervices. Other clinical problems may also be present, such as menorrhagia or pelvic pain; ideally, these should not be dealt with within the context of the colposcopy clinic.

Using a structured format allows important items of data to be captured on all patients, and also allows the transfer of such information to electronic media for storage and analysis. The use of computers further allows repetitive tasks such as letter writing and appointment scheduling to be done automatically, and also allows fail-safe mechanisms to be built into the system (such as routinely flagging missing results, highlighting invasive histology, etc.). Electronic technology also allows for networking, thus bringing together the laboratories, clinic and primary care agencies such as the Family Health Service Authority (FHSA) who operate the recall system.

BASIC MINIMUM DATASET

Whichever system is employed – from the most basic to the most advanced – it is important to adopt a basic minimum dataset. The British Society of Colposcopy and Cervical Pathology (BSCCP) has constructed a basic minimum dataset which forms the basis for personal audit (re-certification), service audit and also national quality control returns.

PERSONAL AUDIT

As part of the certification and recertification process in colposcopy, the BSCCP now asks its practising members to perform regular audits of their own practice. The process is now at its first re-certification stage, and the audit targets are contained within the BSCCP minimum dataset, thereby making it a useful personal audit tool.

REGIONAL AND NATIONAL QUALITY ASSURANCE

The Department of Health will be introducing a statutory return that will require data to be collected by all colposcopy units within primary and secondary trusts in England. This audit form (KC65) will be distributed from the regional quality assurance reference centres. These centres have the responsibility of assessing and maintaining standards of care throughout their regions.

THE KC65 AUDIT FORM

This form is made up of six parts (Figures 9.1–9.6). Its completion and return is mandatory, and therefore there is an obligation of trusts to ensure that this function takes place. Normally, this will be devolved to the lead clinician in colposcopy. The data elements on this form are also largely based upon the BSCCP minimum dataset.

THE BSCCP MINIMUM DATASET

A minimum dataset ensures conformity in the collection of data, allowing measurement against specific standards. Variables to be collected are agreed and defined precisely. The values of these variables should also be defined so that reports from individual clinics can be merged to provide a national picture.

The dataset should use event-based files (i.e. one record for each date on which an event occurred). The dataset is designed based on computerized records systems, but is also compatible with paper usage.

The dataset described is a minimum dataset, and many clinical units will wish to collect more data or more detail. However, local datasets collecting additional data should code down to the minimum dataset to ensure uniformity of data

DH FORM COLPOSCOPY CLINICS: REFERRALS, TREATMENTS AND OUTCOMES   KC65

Quarter ending 30 June 2000   (1)

NHS Trust Name _____   NHS Trust Code R ☐ ☐   (2)

Name of contact _____

Telephone   _____

If you have any queries regarding completion of this form, please contact SD2B

Telephone: 020 7972 5697
                     020 7972 5543

Fax: 020 7972 5662

Return (via Regional QA co-ordinator) to: Department of Health
Statistics Division 2B
Room 430B
Skipton House
Elephant and Castle
London
SE1 6LH

For NHS use. Please use this space to record anything relevant to the quality or consistency of the data.

I confirm that these data are, to the best of my knowledge, an accurate representation of the results obtained from the colposcopy procedures carried out at this trust.

Signed _____   Date _____

Head Clinician

Figure 9.1 The KC65 Audit Form (Colposcopy Clinics – Referrals, Treatments and Outcomes): Front page. (Reproduced with permission of the Department of Health.)

DH FORM PART [A]   Women referred to colposcopy by referral indication and result of referral   [KC65]

(1)		(2)	(3)	(4)	(5)	(6)	(7)	(8)	(9)	(10)	(11)
					Result of referral smear						
Line No.	Referral Indication	Inadequate (cat. 1)	Borderline changes (cat. 8)	Mild dyskaryosis (cat. 3)	Moderate dyskaryosis (cat. 7)	Severe dyskaryosis (cat. 4)	Severe dyskaryosis/ ?Invasive carcinoma (cat. 5)	?Glandular neoplasia (cat. 6)	Other	No referral smear	Total number referred
0001	Screening smear										
0002	Clinical indication										
0003	Total										

Basis: Based on event = 1st appointment in the quarter (regardless of whether woman attended)
ie visit number (MDS item) = 1 and visit description (MDS item) = "new patient attended" or "new patient defaulted"

References: Referral indication (MDS item) [note: line 0002 other = referral indication "abnormal smear after colposcopy",
"clinically suspicious cervix", "suspicious symptoms" or "other"]
Result of Referral smear (MDS item) [note: col 9 other = result "?glandular neoplasia" or "moderate dyskaryosis"]

Figure 9.2 The KC65 Audit Form (Colposcopy Clinics – Referrals, Treatments and Outcomes): Part A. (Reproduced with permission of the Department of Health.)

DH FORM   PART B Women referred to colposcopy by result of referral smear and time from referral to first appointment   KC65

(1)		(2)	(3)	(4)	(5)	(6)	(7)	(8)
			Result of referral smear					
Line No.	Time from referral to first appointment	Inadequate (cat. 1)	Borderline changes/ Mild dyskaryosis (cat. 8/3)	Moderate/ Severe dyskaryosis (cat. 7/4)	Severe/ ?Invasive carcinoma/ ?Glandular neoplasia (cat. 5/6)	Other	Clinical Indication	Total number referred
0001	Less than or equal to 2 weeks							
0002	>2 weeks up to 4 weeks							
0003	>4 weeks up to 8 weeks							
0004	>8 weeks up to 12 weeks							
0005	Over 12 weeks							
0006	Total							

Basis: Based on event = 1st appointment in the quarter (regardless of whether woman attended)
ie visit number (MDS item) = 1 and visit description (MDS item) = "new patient attended" or "new patient defaulted"

References: Result of Referral smear (MDS item)

Time from referral to first appointment = Visit date (MDS item) – Referral date sent (MDS item)
in days: <=14 days
         >14<=28
         >28<=56
         >56<=84
         >84

Note: Referral date sent is date on referral letter or, where direct referral from cytology laboratory, date the smear was reported

Referral indication (MDS item) = "abnormal screening smear" for cols (2)–(5)
                                = any other value for cols (6)–(7)

Figure 9.3 The KC65 Audit Form (Colposcopy Clinics – Referrals, Treatments and Outcomes): Part B. (Reproduced with permission of the Department of Health.)

DH FORM   PART [C]   First attendances by type of procedure and result of referral   [KC65]

(1)	(2)	(3)	(4)	(5)	(6)	(7)
			Procedure type			
			Treatment biopsy or treatment/diagnostic biopsy			
Line No.	Result of referral smear	No treatment	Diagnostic biopsy (punch)	Ablation	Excision	Other	Number of first attendances
0001	Inadequate (cat. 1)						
0002	Borderline changes (cat. 8)						
0003	Mild dyskaryosis (cat. 3)						
0004	Moderate dyskaryosis (cat. 7)						
0005	Severe dyskaryosis (cat. 4)						
0006	Severe dyskaryosis ?Invasive carcinoma (cat. 5)						
0007	?Glandular neoplasia (cat. 6)						
0008	Other						
0009	Clinical indication, no referral smear						
0010	Total						

Basis: Based on event = 1st attendance, occurring in the quarter ie Visit description (MDS item) = new patient attended

References: Treatment type is a combination of MDS items Biopsy type (BT) and Treatment method (TM)
col (2): TM = "no treatment" and BT = "no biopsy"; col (3): TM = "no treatment" and BT = "directed biopsy" or "multiple directed biopsy"
and BT = any other than "no biopsy"; col (5): TM = "loop/laser excision" or "knife cone" and BT = any other than "no biopsy"; col (6): TM = "hysterectomy" or
"other" and BT = any other than "no biopsy"

Result of Referral smear (MDS item) [note: line 0008 other = result "adenocarcinoma" or "abnormal unclassifiable"]

Figure 9.4 The KC65 Audit Form (Colposcopy Clinics – Referrals, Treatments and Outcomes): Part C. (Reproduced with permission of the Department of Health.)

DH FORM   PART D   Biopsies, by time from biopsy to informing patient of result   KC65

(1) Line No.	Waiting times	(2) Total number of biopsies in first month of quarter
0001	Less than or equal to 2 weeks	
0002	>2 weeks up to 4 weeks	
0003	>4 weeks up to 8 weeks	
0004	>8 weeks up to 12 weeks	
0005	Over 12 weeks	
0006	Total	

Basis: Based on event = any attendance at which biopsy type (MDS item) is not "No Biopsy"

Waiting time is "Date patient is informed" (not an MDS item) – Visit date (MDS item)

in days: <=14 days
          >14<=28
          >28<=56
          >56<=84
          >84

Note: (1) As date patient informed is not an MDS item, this part is suited to a retrospective audit, possibly by the QA team, of the date on the information letters sent to patients.

(2) Return to be based on sample of events occurring in 1st month of quarter

Figure 9.5 The KC65 Audit Form (Colposcopy Clinics – Referrals, Treatments and Outcomes): Part D. (Reproduced with permission of the Department of Health.)

PART E   Biopsies by type and outcome

KC65

(1) Line No.	Outcome (Histology result)	(2) Biopsy type Diagnostic (punch)	(3) Biopsy type Other	(4) Total biopsies in first month of quarter
0001	Cancer (including micro-invasive)			
0002	Adenocarcinoma in situ			
0003	CIN3			
0004	CIN2			
0005	CIN1			
0006	HPV/cervicitus only			
0007	No CIN/No HPV (normal)			
0008	Inadequate/unsatisfactory biopsy			
0009	Result not known by clinic			
0010	Total			

Basis: Based on event = any attendance at which biopsy type (MDS item) is not "No Biopsy"

References: Biopsy type (MDS item)
Histology (MDS item)

Note: (1) Histopathology categories to be same as adopted in NHSCSP publication no. 10
(2) To allow time for follow up, record outcome only for biopsies taken in 1st month of quarter

Figure 9.6 The KC65 Audit Form (Colposcopy Clinics – Referrals, Treatments and Outcomes): Part E. (Reproduced with permission of the Department of Health.)

collection. The BSCPP executive, in consultation with the NHSCSP, should decide on changes to the minimum dataset.

In general terms, the following data should be collected:

Referral data

To ensure adequate maintenance of skills:

- The number of new cases managed by individual colposcopists per year
- For training units, the number of cases where trainees are directly supervised by individual colposcopists per year
- The status of the colposcopist
- Trained and accredited (BSCCP)
- Not accredited
- Trainee under supervision
- Trainee, not under supervision
- Other

A 'new case' is defined as a referral generated by an agency separate from the colposcopy provider that is not currently being reviewed by that colposcopy provider. These agencies will usually be primary care-based, but in some situations could be direct referral from the cytology service.

Demographic data

To determine range of patients seen and reason for referral to colposcopy clinic:

- Provider Unit Number and/or NHS number
- Patient's last name*
- Patient's initial*
- Patient's date of birth
- Provider Unit ID
- Referral indication
    Abnormal screening smear
    Abnormal smear, previous colposcopy
    Clinically suspicious cervix
    Suspicious symptoms
    Other

*If relevant

Whilst not considered a part of the minimum dataset, these are considered optional for those units who may also wish to use the dataset for clinic management purposes (i.e. sending letters).

Attendance data

To ensure adequate timeliness of diagnosis.

To measure the waiting time for colposcopic assessment for all referrals; number of days from receipt of referral letter to date of first appointment (whether seen or not) by referral smear:

- Referral smear
  - Severe and moderate dyskaryosis
  - Mild dyskaryosis and borderline
- Referral date received by the colposcopy service
- Referral date sent

Event data

The following data are collected at each colposcopy clinic/operating theatre visit.

To determine the default rate:

- Attended/defaulted (this is a patient-initiated non-attendance)
- Visit date (date that the appointment was scheduled)
- Visit number
- Colposcopist's name
- Colposcopist's status

The following data are obtained from the colposcopic examination in order to ensure quality and accuracy of the diagnosis; they contain an accurate recording of cervical or vaginal colposcopic findings:

- Cytology result
- Visibility of squamocolumnar junction
- Colposcopic opinion of lesion

Cervical	Vaginal*
Normal	Normal
HPV/Inflammation/	HPV/Inflammation/
Other benign changes	Other benign changes
CIN/Low grade	VaIN/Low grade
CIN/High grade	VaIN/High grade
Invasion	Invasion
Other	Other
Not performed	Not performed
No cervix	

*If relevant

The percentage of women at their first visit having a cervical biopsy or a loop excision cross-referenced against a referral smear, and the proportion treated under local anaesthetic:

- Biopsy type
  - Directed/Punch
  - Excisional
  - None

- Treatment method
  - Not treated
  - Ablation
  - Excision
  - Hysterectomy
  - Other

- Analgesia
  - None
  - Local
  - General

- Histology result (three fields are reserved for histology results to enable two cervical histologies and one vaginal histology to be recorded for each attendance).

Values for pathology should be the same for all histological specimens sent, and should correspond to those detailed in Table 9.1. Only one value should be recorded for the same pathology. The highest grades of histological abnormality should be recorded; for example, if CIN1 and CIN2 are both on the pathology report, then only CIN2 should be recorded. If there are two distinct pathologies (not just different grades) in one specimen, for example CIN3 and CGIN in a LLETZ specimen, then two values should be recorded.

Follow-up data

To ensure quality of treatment and adequacy of follow-up:

- As a follow-up visit is 'an event', the date, cytology and histology (if any) will be recorded. Hence, the dataset should be able to output follow-up information based on these data fields.

Table 9.1 Histological categories for cervical and vaginal biopsies

Cervix	Vagina
Unsatisfactory	Unsatisfactory
Normal (including HPV and cervicitis)	Normal (including HPV and cervicitis)
CIN1	VaIN1
CIN2	VaIN2
CIN3	VaIN3
Invasive squamous (Ia_1)	Invasive vaginal carcinoma
Invasive squamous (Ia_2)	Other
Invasive squamous (>Ia)	
CGIN (low-grade)	
CGIN (high-grade)	
Invasive adenocarcinoma	
Other	

CIN, cervical intraepithelial neoplasia; CGIN, cervical glandular intraepithelial neoplasia; HPV, human papillomavirus; VaIN, vaginal intraepithelial neoplasia.

Communications data

To ensure that women and primary carers are adequately informed about treatment:

- The percentage of letters sent in less than 15 working days from the clinic, communicating either results or management plans to the women and their primary carers.

Very few of the electronic systems currently in place in colposcopy clinics will have the facility to easily record the date that letters were sent out to patients following a colposcopy clinic visit. It is suggested that this information may be acquired through regular and random audits of colposcopy clinic letters generated by the colposcopy service.

DATA COLLECTION

The mechanism of collection and subsequent analysis must be robust if the data are to serve as a reliable record. There are many different methods of data collection and analysis, and individual clinics will be able to choose one that will suit their own circumstances.

Clinics may already use electronic data collection. If so, users will need to ensure that the data fields that comprise the minimum dataset are included in their databases, and preferably be able to generate outputs that are compatible with 'a standard annual return' based on the minimum dataset. Those planning to purchase systems should ensure that the system will collect the data required. An alternative may be a 'Bureau' system, whereby the user collects the dataset information on a standard form and sends this to an external agency ('Bureau') which transcribes the data into an electronic format. The Bureau then stores the information electronically and produces reports for the user at predefined intervals.

RECORDING THE COLPOSCOPIC IMAGE

REASONS FOR RECORDING IMAGES

The main reason for recording colposcopic images is so that comparison may be made at future visits, especially when the decision is to observe the condition rather than treat. A second reason is for audit purposes, and this is particularly the case when the colposcopist is on a learning curve and trying to match their colposcopic expertise with histological outcome. Each of these reasons is sufficient in its own right to demand some form of recording. Again, there is a wide variation in recording techniques and accuracy.

IMAGE RECORDING TECHNIQUES

The most widely used – but least accurate – method is a simple hand drawing. Unfortunately, these are usually not to scale, they only record the presence or absence of a lesion, and may also specify whether or not the whole transformation zone (TZ) was visualized. A fairly good example of a hand-drawn recording of a colposcopic assessment is shown in Figure 9.7. This particular schematic illustrates that the colposcopist could see the whole TZ, has identified a significant lesion within it, and has also identified that some areas may be worse than others (although as both are pre-invasive this would not alter the treatment strategy). Had atypical vessels or an irregular surface contour been documented, then a colposcopic opinion of early invasion might have been made.

The shortcomings of this method are that it is difficult to quantify the size of the abnormality, and it is wholly subjective and difficult to reproduce. The former problem can be partly addressed by attempting to semiquantitate the lesion. This can be done by superimposing imaginary lines on the image so as to divide the

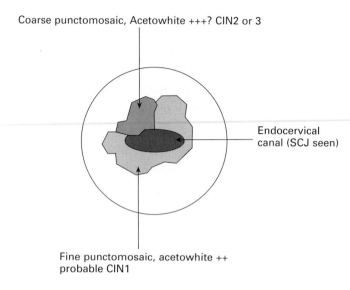

Coarse punctomosaic, Acetowhite +++? CIN2 or 3

Endocervical
canal (SCJ seen)

Fine punctomosaic, acetowhite ++
probable CIN1

Figure 9.7 Diagrammatic representation of colposcopic abnormalities.

cervix into 'measurement sectors' (Figure 9.8). First, a circle is drawn on the cervix with its centre at the middle of the external os and its radius reaching to a point midway between the external os and the cervicovaginal junction (line A). A second line bisects the cervix laterally (line B) and a third anteroposteriorly (line C). In this way, the cervix is divided into eight sectors (see Figure 9.8). There are consistent data linking large surface-area lesions with high-grade histology, and also an increased likelihood of treatment failure.

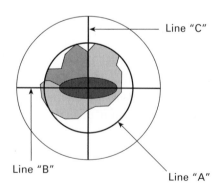

Line "C"

Line "B"

Line "A"

Figure 9.8 Schematic of a '5-sector' lesion.

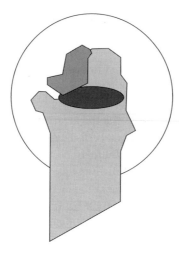

Figure 9.9 Lesion extending on to the posterior fornix.

Freehand drawing is also used to illustrate abnormalities at the vaginal vault. If the cervix is still in place, this is usually represented by just extending the area of abnormality on to the vagina, as indicated in Figure 9.9.

Sometimes, after a hysterectomy for pre-invasive disease a woman may persist in having – or may develop – abnormal vaginal vault smears, and this might indicate vaginal intraepithelial neoplasia (VaIN). In this situation the vaginal vault is usually pictured as in Figure 9.10. The transverse line represents the vaginal vault scar, whilst the angled lines at either end represent the vaginal angles. This is not very satisfactory, as the vaginal angles can be deeply pocketed following hysterectomy and the schematic cannot account for this.

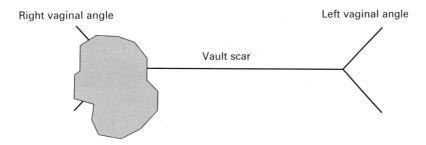

Figure 9.10 Lesion involving the right vaginal angle and the vaginal vault scar.

OTHER METHODS OF IMAGE CAPTURE AND STORAGE

COLPOPHOTOGRAPHY

Photography offers an obvious solution to the problem of subjectivity and accuracy. Most colposcopes will allow for the attachment of a beam-splitting device so that the image seen by the colposcopist can be diverted to a fixed camera, without altering the image seen. There is usually some loss of light intensity however. The camera is attached directly to the beam-splitter and no lens adjustments are necessary once the equipment has been set up. The film used is 35 mm colour film (usual speed ASA 200), with flash exposure on an f16/32 aperture setting. Using this set-up limits the depth of focus, which is the major problem of colpophotography. Black and white film is preferred, with the addition of a green filter if the subepithelial capillary architecture is to be emphasized (good for atypical vessels). A flash device may be used: a ring flash around the colposcope objective lens is useful in this situation.

Photographs may also be taken without the use of the colposcope. Hand-held cameras must be used at higher shutter speeds in order to compensate for shake. Again, a flash device is necessary and in addition some alternative light source to illuminate the cervix to enable the target shot to be focused properly. The quality of these photographs is generally inferior to those taken with the aid of the colposcope.

A further development of photography was the introduction of the cerviscope. This consists of a 35-mm camera body, a 50-mm extension ring, and a 100-mm macrolens with a ring stroboscopic light. This in effect is a customized camera of fixed focal length that takes 35-mm exposures under enhanced illumination and flash capacity. Since the exposure time is determined by the duration of the flash of the strobe light (<1/2000th of a second), hand vibrations of the person holding the cerviscope will not affect the quality of the slides. The device was primarily intended as a substitute for colposcopy (in areas where no colposcopy was available). The exposures taken are sent for expert analysis (by projection and analysis at a fixed distance from the screen), thus enabling selection of those women who would require colposcopy and biopsy.

All the above photographic methods of image capture have similar drawbacks:

- The image is not immediately available for scrutiny; therefore the eventual quality of the image cannot be assessed.
- The cervix is a three-dimensional structure, whereas colpophotographs are not (even with enhanced depth of focus, this is a potential shortcoming).

- Transparencies are a less than ideal method of storing image data alongside other data.
- It is relatively expensive.
- Once collected, the image cannot be enhanced, magnified or annotated.

VIDEOCOLPOSCOPY

Modern video cameras are small and produce high-quality images (particularly three-chip cameras). These can also be attached, via a beam-splitting device, to a standard colposcope. Many clinics routinely employ video for patient information purposes (although not all patients wish to observe procedures), and for teaching. Because video offers a time dimension as well as the image, several different views of the same cervix are possible and can all be stored. Views include different magnifications, addition of green filters, before and after the application of saline, acetic acid or iodine. One video, therefore, can contain the same information as multiple still exposures. This does not remove the problem of depth of focus, but it does allow a more comprehensive assessment.

Video images can be stored either on tape or disc. The former approach is both bulky and inconvenient in terms of recall, whilst the latter only suffers from problems of memory, i.e. video images require large amounts of computer storage such that one standard 3.5-inch floppy disc can only store three or four compressed video images. Compact disc offers greater scope for image storage, but it is more expensive.

Images captured by video cameras are digitized signals, and utilizing this approach allows for both storage and image manipulation. Some colposcopy clinics already employ digitized image capture, storage and analysis, and it is proving to be a useful teaching, audit and research tool. Whether it actually enhances clinical care is debatable, however.

The computer's storage, analysis and manipulation systems allow the images to be instantly recalled, to be compared with previously recalled images, and to be enhanced in terms of contrast, sharpness and brightness. Additionally, electronic filters can be employed to enhance selectively the vasculature and acetowhiteness. As the image is stored, it can also be measured electronically (area, perimeter), thus dispensing with the need for semiquantitative measurements. A printed (hard) copy of the image can be produced to store alongside the patient's written record or, alternatively, the written information can be stored in a database alongside the stored image, allowing for a complete set of electronic notes.

Few clinics have this capacity as yet, and it is arguable that few will actually need this high degree of data management. Nevertheless, a structured and meticulous approach to data management in the colposcopy clinic, be it hand-written structured case notes or direct-entry computerized notes, is and will continue to be an important aspect of work in the colposcopy clinic. Hence, it is a discipline that should be acquired by all practising colposcopists.

LEARNING POINTS

- Accurate recording of the information gained at colposcopy is an important aspect of service provision.
- Minimum datasets are essential for personal and national audit.
- Minimum datasets need not record information on previous sexual history unless this is part of an ethically agreed protocol, or is part of a genitourinary medicine service.
- Electronic storage of information will allow for the automation of repetitive tasks such as appointment scheduling and communication with referring agencies. It will also allow fail-safes to be built into the system to track invasive cancers, defaulting patients, etc.
- Image recording is useful for making comparisons at further clinic visits. The simplest methods, such as hand-drawings, are also the least objective.
- Objective image-capturing techniques include various photographic and videocolposcopic techniques.

MCQs

For answers to Questions, see Appendix C.

24. **Recording information in colposcopy clinics:**
    a. The number of previous sexual partners is an essential part of the colposcopy minimum dataset.
    b. The minimum dataset records the findings of bimanual examination at the first attendance.
    c. Photography is useful in assessing the extent of involvement of the vaginal angles in VaIN.
    d. The patient's hospital number is the preferred unique identifier.
    e. The use of digital image capture has no proven benefits in managing patients in the colposcopy clinic.

25. **In colpophotography:**
    a. A beam-splitting device attached to the colposcopes reduces the light intensity.
    b. Black and white film (enhanced by the addition of a red filter) is better for recording vascular architecture.
    c. Videophotography gives better depth of focus than still photography.
    d. Cervicographs are assessed by an expert, who examines the projected slide of the cervix at a fixed distance.
    e. A film speed of 400 ASA is ideal for photographing the cervix.

chapter 10

CONSERVATIVE MANAGEMENT OF CIN

M.I. Shafi

INTRODUCTION

There is a large discrepancy between the number of women with abnormal cervical cytology and those developing invasive cervical cancer. Mortality associated with cervical cancer continues to fall in the United Kingdom, and is associated with high coverage of the at-risk population. The most recent data suggest that the extent of such coverage is 84%.

Among cervical smears, 8.3% demonstrate some form of abnormality. The majority of patients have only minor cytological abnormalities, and only a small percentage would develop cancer. The invasive potential of cervical intraepithelial neoplasia (CIN) has long been known, but trying to quantify the risk overall – and especially for the individual woman – is fraught with difficulties. In some studies, the progression rates are extremely high, with almost all high-grade lesions progressing to invasive cancer, whilst in others only a small minority will progress. What is known is that the more severe the cytological abnormality, the higher the risk of finding invasive disease when the woman is assessed. Similarly, a group of women with a histological diagnosis of CIN3 are more likely to progress than a group of women with CIN1 or HPV-associated changes only. This does not help in predicting for the individual woman her risk for progression from CIN to invasive cancer, however. Based partly on these facts, the Royal College of Obstetricians and Gynaecologists (RCOG) recommendations in 1987 stated that all grades of CIN should undergo treatment. More recently, it has been realized that this policy has led to overtreatment for many women, especially with the introduction of a 'see-and-treat' management strategy using large loop excision of the transformation zone (LLETZ). In reviewing the evidence, the national guidelines were changed in 1992 to state that CIN1 may be treated or kept under close surveillance.

HOW DO WE SELECT PATIENTS?

In many units the women are assessed in colposcopy units, and colposcopically directed punch biopsies are taken from the worst area of abnormality. Dependent upon the results of this investigation, the woman is either offered treatment or observation as indicated. For the high-grade lesions (CIN2 and 3), immediate treatment should be conducted, but for the low-grade lesions (CIN1 or human papillomavirus (HPV)-associated changes), treatment may be offered or a deferred management strategy may be adopted depending on the circumstances. For example, in a woman who is aged 45 years and has completed her family, a punch biopsy diagnosis of CIN1 is likely to lead to treatment. In contrast, a woman in her early 20s who has the same diagnosis but is nulliparous and has only a small area of abnormality may be offered a conservative management option in the hope that the lesion will regress over time and both colposcopic assessment and cervical cytology will return to normal.

In some centres, it is normal practice not to take any diagnostic punch biopsies prior to treatment. In these units, a colposcopic diagnosis on the grounds of abnormal cervical cytology is deemed sufficient, but this is affected by the subjective nature of colposcopic assessment. There may be considerable inter- as well as intra-observer disagreement in relation to the colposcopic findings. These units mostly practise excisional forms of treatment (LLETZ, laser excision) and the excised transformation zone is sent for histological diagnosis. Some women will not require treatment, including those who have abnormal cervical cytology and no colposcopic abnormality. In such women, colposcopic and cytological review should continue until at least two negative smears are obtained 6 months apart before they are discharged back to the general practitioner. In those women deemed to have a low-grade lesion on colposcopic assessment, a deferred management strategy may be adopted only if the colposcopist is confident of the diagnosis. Treatment should be offered if the lesion deteriorates either because the cytology shows more severe changes or because colposcopically the lesion appears worse (for example, the size of the lesion increases or stigmata of high-grade disease, such as coarse mosaicism, become apparent). Not taking a colposcopically directed biopsy may be perceived as an inaccurate science, but so could taking a directed biopsy from the wrong area of a lesion. Those with sufficient experience are normally happy to rely on the colposcopic assessment for those women thought to have a low-grade lesion, as review cytology and colposcopy will identify any progression of the lesion.

HISTOLOGICAL INTERPRETATION

While taking a punch biopsy would seem judicious if there is concern about the diagnosis, one must be aware that histological interpretation is not without problems. Although there is generally good agreement at the higher end of the CIN spectrum, this is not the case at the lower end when trying to differentiate CIN1 and HPV-associated changes. There is also a tendency to overcall low-grade lesions on punch biopsy, leading to unnecessary treatment. Further bias may be introduced if the colposcopist does not sample the worst area of colposcopic abnormality.

PROGRESSIVE POTENTIAL OF CIN

The pathological spectrum of CIN has been arbitrarily divided into three grades: 1, 2 and 3 (see Chapter 3). These grades are associated with a different risk of progressive potential, and have recently been revised to high-grade lesions (CIN2 and 3) that are likely to be cancer precursors, and low-grade lesions (CIN1 and HPV-associated changes) that have unknown but probable low risk of progressive potential. The progressive potential of CIN is also likely to be related to the size of the lesion as well as its grade. For example, a large CIN3 lesion would be expected to have a higher risk of progression than a small focus of CIN3 surrounded by a low-grade lesion. Despite this, there is unanimity that once CIN3 is diagnosed, treatment should be offered. An exception to this would be in the pregnant woman, where treatment may need to be deferred (see Chapter 15).

DEFERRED MANAGEMENT

If a decision is made between the colposcopist and the woman to defer treatment for a low-grade lesion, then sufficient stress needs to be placed on the need for continued colposcopic and cytological surveillance. If there is any likelihood of non-compliance, then treatment should be offered. For those women willing to comply, both colposcopy and cytology should be repeated at 6-monthly intervals. If the abnormality persists either colposcopically or cytologically (usually an arbitrary upper limit of 24 months is set), then treatment should be offered. If the lesion regresses, the surveillance is continued until two consecutive smears are negative, at which point the woman may be returned to the 3-yearly screening programme.

THE PROBLEM OF DEFAULT

This is an area of considerable concern in those women undergoing deferred management. In two recent prospective studies examining the management of minor cytological abnormalities, the cumulative default rate was approximately 20%, though depending on the catchment area of the colposcopy clinic this may be as high as 30%. If there is a problem of default from clinics in those women selected for deferred management, then this policy is not sustainable and should be abandoned for a more pragmatic approach. If, however, default rates are low with a stable population, a selective policy of deferred management can be safely undertaken without prejudicing the long-term prognosis for the woman. Mechanisms should exist in all colposcopy clinics to limit the problem of default. Such measures could include better communication; a better clinic environment; explanations as to why compliance is important; clinic times that are suitable for women with varying commitments (e.g. evening clinics) and appropriate counselling. A key element is that all advice given to the women should be the same irrespective of the source, and in this respect written instructions and advice are extremely useful (see Chapter 17).

HPV TESTING

As HPV is found in the vast majority of invasive cervical cancers, testing for the oncogenic types may hold potential for increased diagnostic and management accuracy in women presenting with abnormal cervical cytology. In cross-sectional studies, the presence of oncogenic HPV virus types predicts with good sensitivity and specificity the presence of high-grade intraepithelial disease that would require treatment. The major role for HPV testing may be in women over the age of 35 years, as it is the persistence of the HPV infection that is linked to the development of cervical cancer. In those women with equivocal cervical smear abnormalities, HPV testing may be used to identify those women requiring colposcopy and possible treatment as opposed to those that can safely be monitored using cytological and HPV surveillance. This is particularly the case with liquid-based cytology (LBC) where the HPV testing can be undertaken on the same specimen used for cytological assessment. Using this approach should minimize unnecessary investigations in the colposcopy clinic.

SUMMARY

While the conservative option in the management of CIN is not suitable for all cases, it is certainly one to consider if any impact is to be made on the overtreatment potential of a 'see-and-treat' strategy. This is particularly the case for younger women with low-grade lesions, as many of these will regress over time. During any conservative management strategy, the importance of compliance with the surveillance programme cannot be overstressed. The management algorithm (Figure 10.1) summarizes a conservative approach to the management of mildly

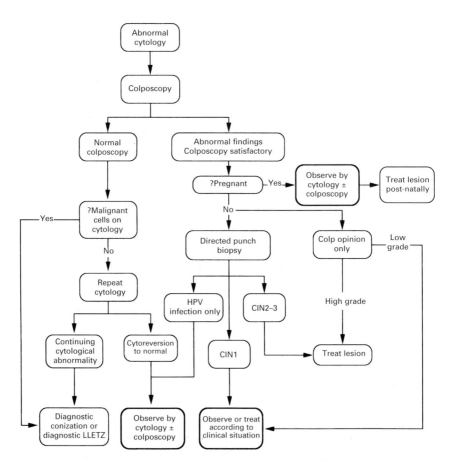

Figure 10.1 Flow chart for management of women with cytological abnormalities. (Reproduced with permission from *RCOG Yearbook*, 1995, RCOG Press.)

abnormal smears. The use of HPV testing as an adjunct to cervical cytology continues to be the subject of study.

LEARNING POINTS

- Not all cases of CIN will progress to invasive cancer.
- High-grade CIN is known to have malignant potential, whereas low-grade lesions have unknown malignant potential.
- Accurate colposcopic assessment and appropriate directed biopsies are necessary for those women considered suitable for conservative management.
- High-grade lesions should be treated once diagnosed.
- Low-grade lesions can either be treated or kept under close surveillance.
- Default rates should be considered when deciding whether a woman may be conservatively managed.

CLINICAL CASE SCENARIO 3

A 22-year-old nulliparous woman attended for her first ever cervical smear. She enjoyed good general health and had no gynaecological symptoms. The cervical smear was reported as showing mildly dyskaryotic changes.

Questions

1. Should this woman be referred for immediate colposcopic assessment?
2. Follow-up showed mild dyskaryosis and colposcopy was consistent with HGCIN. Should the patient undergo immediate LLETZ?
3. Following treatment is the woman at increased risk of invasive cervical cancer?

MCQs

For answers to Questions, see Appendix C.

26. **Epidemiology:**
    a. The incidence of cervical cancer continues to decline.
    b. Cervical cancer is the commonest female cancer worldwide.
    c. Approximately 11% of all cervical smears taken are abnormal to some degree.

d. Almost 10% of smears taken in the UK are reported as unsatisfactory.

e. Almost 6 million smears are performed annually in the UK.

27. **Patient selection:**
    a. All cases of CIN must undergo immediate treatment.
    b. A colposcopic-directed punch biopsy should always be taken in women with abnormal cervical cytology.
    c. A colposcopic-directed punch biopsy can be helpful in assessing the degree of abnormality.
    d. High-grade CIN in pregnancy should be immediately treated.
    e. Young women with low-grade CIN may be managed conservatively.

28. **Non-treatment of cytological abnormalities:**
    a. If there is no lesion present at colposcopy, the woman should be discharged to routine screening.
    b. Women with CIN3 have a lower progressive potential than those with CIN1.
    c. HPV testing may predict those women with high-grade CIN.
    d. HPV testing may allow selection of those women requiring colposcopy among those with equivocal cytological abnormalities.
    e. CIN has a centripetal distribution (i.e. higher-grade CIN is centrally placed in a lesion).

chapter 11

TREATMENT METHODS AND HOW TO SELECT

D.M. Luesley

INTRODUCTION

Any screening programme must have as one of its components an intervention that is both timely and effective in preventing the natural progression of disease. In cervical intraepithelial neoplasia (CIN), this intervention or treatment occurs following the cytological, colposcopic and histological recognition of precursors that carry an increased risk of progression to invasive disease.

Not all CIN will become cancer, and there is therefore a need to select cases for treatment on the basis of risk. Once a decision to treat has been made, the most appropriate form of treatment is selected.

WHO REQUIRES TREATMENT?

There is a growing body of opinion, which feels that minor abnormalities (CIN1 with or without koilocytosis or koilocytosis alone) may be observed, as there is a reasonable prospect of spontaneous resolution over time. The critical issue here is one of accurate initial diagnosis. Up to 40% of minor cytological abnormalities will be associated with underlying high-grade disease, and as most (if not all) colposcopists would recommend treatment of high-grade lesions, decisions that rely on cytology alone will significantly underestimate such lesions.

The addition of colposcopy improves the selection process, yet is still not 100% accurate. Even adding directed or targeted biopsies fails to achieve this level of accuracy in diagnosis. Given the inadequacies of our diagnostic procedures we are left in a situation where specificity is sacrificed in favour of sensitivity; that is, it is more acceptable to overtreat a group of women who might never have developed cancer in order not to miss the smaller group who might well progress. This philosophy is possible only because the available treatment modalities are relatively simple, safe and effective. Thus, the treatment methodology itself is a variable that determines the level of intervention. As an example, if the only treatment method available were radical hysterectomy, then the threshold for offering treatment would be much higher. At the other extreme, simple outpatient loop excision – which is quick, safe, cheap and effective – has resulted in a lowering of the intervention threshold, a practice typified by the 'see-and-treat' philosophy.

'SEE-AND-TREAT'

The true 'see-and-treat' approach is one that assumes that all women referred to a colposcopy clinic with an abnormal smear are at an increased risk of developing cancer and are therefore treated by an excisional method at their first attendance to the clinic. The advantages of such an approach are as follows:

- All patients at risk are treated.
- There is a more rapid return to cytological normality.
- All occult cancers will be detected.
- There are fewer visits required and therefore less cost to both the service and the patient.
- Very little (if any) colposcopic expertise is required.

These points may seem convincing, yet this approach leads to excessive intervention. Even though the morbidity associated with loop excision is low it is not nil; therefore unnecessary morbidity will be generated. Some would argue that this type of early and effective intervention would be associated with a lesser degree of psychosocial trauma. This has yet to be confirmed and the converse may also be true; that is, the very act of intervention reinforces the 'disease state'. While many clinics currently do employ a 'see-and-treat' approach, more are adopting the more conservative selective philosophy.

SELECTIVE APPROACH TO TREATMENT

The colposcopist aims to treat only those where there is a reasonable suspicion of high-grade disease. This suspicion is based upon the cytological status, colposcopic appearances of the lesion and, if necessary, targeted biopsies. The aim is to reduce overtreatment, although even with a selective approach some women with either low-grade disease or koilocytotic atypia will still be overtreated. There is also an additional burden of counselling and following up those who have not been treated. A higher level of colposcopic expertise is required and it is less efficient in resource use. As diagnostic acumen improves, and especially as we employ more specific investigations such as human papillomavirus (HPV) subtyping, the selection process will become more refined.

Some of the criteria employed in constructing the treatment algorithm are shown in Figure 11.1.

Cytology and colposcopy follow-up are integral components of a 'select-and-treat' strategy, and although there are no data to suggest how long such a follow-up period should be, an arbitrary figure of 2 years is usually employed. Few women will be happy to undertake further surveillance, particularly if their smear remains abnormal, albeit a minor abnormality. Furthermore, those who have had persistently abnormal smears for this period of time are more likely to have a lesion that will not regress. This, however, is an area for further research.

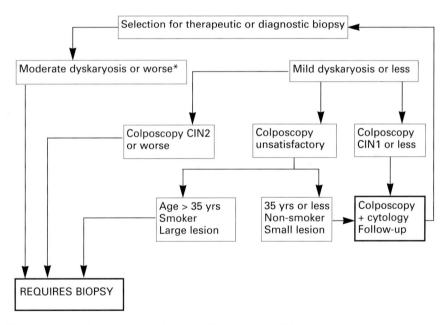

*There may be circumstances where the biopsy can be delayed. In pregnancy, for example, biopsy can be delayed until after delivery unless there is a suspicion of invasive disease. If a biopsy is not taken, the reason for not biopsying should be clearly recorded.

Figure 11.1 Who to select for diagnostic/therapeutic biopsy.

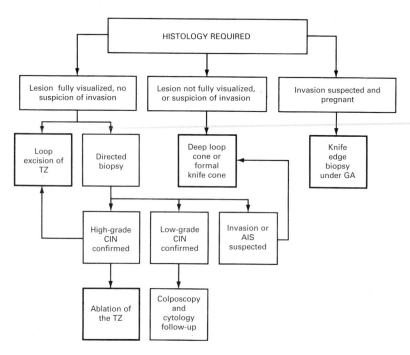

Figure 11.2 Selection of biopsy method.

If, either at the first visit or during subsequent follow-up, the criteria for intervention are met, a further series of decisions based upon the three criteria (cytology, colposcopy and histology) are required (Figure 11.2).

The types of treatment available are many, and individual choices should be matched against specific criteria. Perhaps the most important decision to make at this point is to exclude invasive disease.

A further point that needs to be considered is the relative increase in the proportion of women with minor cytological abnormalities referred for colposcopic assessment. Within this cohort there will undoubtedly be women with high-grade disease, but there will also be a large number with either no disease, transient HPV infections or minor abnormalities that will revert to normal. Treating all of these women does not seem justifiable. In our own practice, 981 new cases referred over 2 years (representing 40% of the total new referrals) had no colposcopically identifiable lesion. In 345 cases the squamocolumnar junction could not be defined. If one also takes into account the severity of the referral smear, well over 75% had mild dyskaryosis or less. A subsequent analysis of women with normal colposcopy and only borderline changes on their referral smear demonstrated that of 295 women, only 23 (7.8%) eventually required treatment. All treatments were prompted by deterioration in cytology, and only one occurred before 18 months. Furthermore, only five women had high-grade disease. In the absence of high-grade cytology, normal colposcopy does not warrant intervention. Persisting mild dyskaryosis certainly requires biopsy, and if there is no obvious lesion then a loop excision of the transformation zone should be considered. Destructive therapy is unwise when colposcopy is normal, as any directed biopsies are by definition random and blind.

EXCLUDING INVASIVE DISEASE

Local destruction or excision are inappropriate methods to manage invasive disease, although some cases of stage Ia_1 and Ia_2 disease can be managed by large cones (knife, loop or laser). Invasive disease should be suspected if:

- Naked eye examination is suspicious.
- Colposcopy is suspicious of invasion (atypical vessels, irregular cervix, etc.)
- Cytological features of invasion (malignant diathesis) are present.
- Malignant glandular cells are seen in the smear.
- The whole transformation zone (TZ) cannot be visualized; in this situation colposcopy is deemed unsatisfactory as there will always be the possibility of an invasive process within the part of the TZ that has not been seen.

If any of these criteria are met, then a large representative biopsy of the whole TZ should be taken. The methods employed to achieve this are:

- knife cone biopsy;
- deep loop cone biopsy; or
- laser cone biopsy.

Most would still favour a knife cone in these situations, as there is less likelihood of damaging the excision margins. Clear interpretation of the excision margins is important for accurate substaging as it is impossible to substage stage Ia cancers unless the whole lesion is seen in the specimen. This may not be possible if there is any degree of thermal artefact obscuring interpretation of the cone edges. If adenocarcinoma-*in-situ* is suspected, the management should be as for suspected invasive disease.

SUSPECTED INVASION IN PREGNANCY

In pregnancy, biopsies are usually avoided because of the increased risk of haemorrhage. They are therefore only performed if there is a high degree of suspicion of an invasive process. This is clearly an area where expert colposcopy is required. In order to minimize cervical trauma and damage, yet still provide adequate histological material to allow an accurate diagnosis of invasion or no invasion, a compromise is made and a wedge of the most atypical part of the TZ is removed under general anaesthesia. This must be regarded as diagnostic only – it is not a form of treatment for invasion or CIN.

THE PRINCIPLES OF TREATING CIN

Several basic principles apply to all forms of treatment.

- If CIN is to be treated, all grades are treated in the same way. High-grade CIN does not require any more radicality than low-grade CIN.
- The whole TZ should be treated or excised, and not just the area where CIN has been identified.
- CIN can – and does – involve gland crypts; therefore any treatment form must address this issue and treat to below the level of gland crypts. A minimum depth of destruction of 7 mm is recommended.
- All treated patients remain at a slightly increased risk of cancer in the future. Cervical cytology follow-up should be offered to all treated patients.

TYPES OF TREATMENT

Many types of treatment are available, and these fall into one of two categories:

1. **Excisional** methods, where the TZ is removed intact and is therefore available for full histological assessment.
2. **Destructive** or **ablative** methods.

When using the latter approach, histological diagnosis must always be obtained by biopsy before treatment is applied. This is the only way to reduce the risk of inadvertently treating invasive disease. Thus, it follows that if a 'see-and-treat' policy is to be used, an excisional form of treatment must be employed (Table 11.1).

Table 11.1 Treatment methods for CIN

Excisional	Destructive
Knife cone biopsy	Cryocautery
Laser cone biopsy	Laser ablation
Loop cone biopsy	Electrodiathermy
Laser or loop TZ excision	Cold coagulation
Hysterectomy	Chemodestruction (5FU, DNCB)

DNCB, dinitrochlorobenzene; 5FU, 5-fluorouracil; TZ, transformation zone.

The difference between a cone biopsy and a TZ excision is largely a matter of degree. Cone biopsy usually refers to a procedure where an attempt is made to remove at least two-thirds of the endocervical canal, and occasionally more. A TZ excision refers to a procedure where the TZ can be seen and the excision process purely aims at obtaining the correct depth (>7 mm) and reasonable clearance (>3 mm) at the edges.

Cryocautery is becoming less popular, largely as a result of published results indicating higher failure rates. This, of course, may not be the fault of the technique but of the operator. Nevertheless, it is probably less effective in achieving the appropriate depth of destruction, and can be difficult to perform with large lesions.

Chemodestructive techniques have been performed, but the long-term outcomes are poor and they are not currently used in clinical practice.

Cold coagulation is really a misnomer. Here, a probe (similar to a cryoprobe) is applied to the cervix, but the tissue is destroyed by heat (>120°C).

Hysterectomy is an effective form of treatment, but is only used if there is an indication for the procedure on its own, i.e. confirmed CIN but also a complaint of menorrhagia or some other problem that would be best managed by hysterectomy. As with the other forms of treatment, it is important to exclude invasion first, as a simple hysterectomy would be inappropriate treatment for invasive disease. Furthermore, if hysterectomy is the chosen method of treatment, colposcopy should accurately delineate the most caudal extension of the TZ in order to include any vaginal extension in a vaginal cuff.

ANALGESIA

Treatment can be performed on an outpatient basis, usually with a local anaesthetic. The cervix is infiltrated with a mixture of a local anaesthetic (lignocaine, prilocaine) and a vasoconstrictor (octapressin or adrenaline). A dental syringe and needle are employed and the cervix is infiltrated to a point where the tissues are seen to blanche. Care should be taken to infiltrate **around** and not into the TZ, as there is a theoretical risk that malignant cells could be introduced deep into the stroma. Local anaesthetics are usually effective in 2 min, and allow most of the outpatient excisional and ablative procedures to be completed with minimal (if any) discomfort to the patient.

The following can be performed as outpatient procedures under local analgesia:

- Laser ablation
- Cold coagulation
- Loop and laser excision
- Cryocautery (though this may be performed without any analgesia).

Some patients will be better treated under a general anaesthetic. It is clear that hysterectomy should be performed under a general anaesthetic, as indeed are most formal knife cone and wedge biopsies. However, about 10% of women will be better managed under a general anaesthetic by one of the outpatient techniques. This is because of patient anxiety or request, or because of poor access to the cervix. In the latter case, better access and control can be achieved in the anaesthetized patient.

COMPLICATIONS OF TREATMENT

IMMEDIATE COMPLICATIONS

Pain and **haemorrhage** are the two problems that are most likely to occur. The former affects very few women now that most treatments are performed under local anaesthetic. Significant haemorrhage, sufficient either to prolong treatment or require remedial measures such as suturing, admission, etc., is quite uncommon (<2% of all cases). In most cases bleeding can be controlled either with the laser or by diathermy. Cold coagulation does not cause primary haemorrhage. There is no reliable way of predicting who will haemorrhage. Obvious infections such as *Trichomonas vaginalis* should be treated before local excision or ablation as they are associated with increased cervical vascularity. It was once thought that treatment should not be performed either during or shortly after menstruation, though apart from the more obvious problems of achieving good visibility, menstruation is not associated with any increased haemorrhagic morbidity.

DELAYED COMPLICATIONS

Secondary haemorrhage can occur at any time up to 14 days after treatment, and is usually the result of a minor infection in the crater where the TZ had existed. This will occur in 1–2% of treated patients. Prophylactic antibiotics are used in some clinics, but their use has not been shown to reduce the frequency of this complication.

Pelvic infection has been reported following local cervical treatment but only on an *ad hoc* basis. There would appear to be an increased risk of this if an intrauterine device is fitted immediately following treatment.

Cervical stenosis (defined as narrowing of the external os to <3 mm) occurs after all methods of treatment. It is much more likely to occur after large conizations, and affects 1–2% of women managed by loop excision of the TZ. The complication is more likely in post-menopausal women. Cervical stenosis may be asymptomatic or cause dysmenorrhoea or, in extreme cases, haematometra. The anatomical distortion of the cervix may make follow-up cervical cytology either difficult or inaccurate, as the new TZ may become inaccessible.

There are no data available confirming that local destruction or excision results in reduced fertility, although this is a natural concern and a theoretical possibility. Neither are there any data suggesting any increase in miscarriage, pre-term labour or failure of the cervix to dilate in labour. Some groups have noted a poorer obstetric performance in treated women, though whether this relates to direct complications of treatment or perhaps to pre-existing factors such as smoking is uncertain. While largely unconfirmed, the concerns over possible impairment of reproductive performance are sufficient to provide support for a more selective approach to treatment.

TREATMENT OUTCOMES

Most methods of treatment have success rates in the order of 95%. Not all patients return to cytological normality within 6 months, but very few – if managed appropriately – will have persisting CIN. The incidence of invasive cancer following local treatments is similar for all methods, including hysterectomy.

CONCLUSIONS

Treatment is an integral part of the programme for the prevention of cervical cancer, and should not be undertaken by anyone other than a trained colposcopist.

With careful selection for treatment and appropriate use of treatment methods, successful outcomes with low morbidity can be achieved.

LEARNING POINTS

- Not all patients with CIN will require treatment, although most with high-grade disease will.
- It is important to exclude invasion prior to local destruction.
- 'See-and-treat' management should only be performed using excisional treatment methods.
- Most methods of local treatment can be performed under local anaesthetic, and have success rates in excess of 90%.
- If there is any suspicion of invasion, then large representative biopsies should be taken.
- Only trained colposcopists should undertake treatment of CIN.
- Hysterectomy is appropriate treatment if there is a specific indication; it does not dispense with the initial need for a thorough colposcopic evaluation.
- Although good data are lacking relating treatment to impaired reproductive performance, there are sufficient concerns to be more selective about treatment.

MCQs

For answers to Questions, see Appendix C.

29. **In the treatment of CIN:**
    a. Excision and ablation are both appropriate in recurrent cases.
    b. All methods other than hysterectomy require prior colposcopy.
    c. Before ablation, a directed biopsy should be performed.
    d. Loop excision can be used to 'see-and-treat' without recourse to biopsy.
    e. Local anaesthetic is injected into the TZ prior to excision.

30. **The following situations require a biopsy:**
    a. Mild dyskaryosis in a 22-year-old with normal satisfactory colposcopy.
    b. Two borderline smears in a 28-year-old previously treated for CIN2.
    c. Suspected CIN1 in pregnancy.
    d. Cervical smear in a 40-year-old reported as glandular atypia.
    e. Mild dyskaryosis in a 60-year-old with leukoplakia on the cervix.

31. **Treatment of CIN should not be performed:**
   a. In pregnancy.
   b. If there is an acute vaginal infection.
   c. In the luteal phase.
   d. During menstruation.
   e. In women who are HIV-positive.

chapter 12

FOLLOW-UP AFTER COLPOSCOPY

H.C. Kitchener

INTRODUCTION

Appropriate follow-up is an essential part of any colposcopy management protocol. The purpose of this chapter is to explain the need for follow-up in both treated and untreated patients. The methods of follow-up which should be employed and for how long will also be discussed. Colposcopic examination is employed in a variety of clinical situations:

- As the initial means of diagnosis following an abnormal smear.
- As a means of selective ablation or excision of the transformation zone.
- As a means of follow-up after treatment of cervical intraepithelial neoplasia (CIN).
- Continued surveillance following an inconclusive initial examination.

THE NEED FOR FOLLOW-UP AFTER TREATMENT OF CIN

The reasons why follow-up is so important following treatment are three-fold:

1. To ensure that there is no residual CIN, or even cancer.
2. To ensure that any recurrence of CIN is detected.
3. To ensure that there have been no clinical problems since treatment.

In order to design the most effective follow-up protocol it is necessary to have an understanding both of the risks of treatment failure and of longer-term recurrence of both CIN and cancer. The more rigorous the follow-up protocol, the less likely that treatment failure will go unrecognized. On the other hand, a more intensive protocol will consume more clinical resources, and women may be made to experience continued anxiety. For some women the process of treatment is not over until discharge from the colposcopy clinic, and until that time there may be continued concern.

TREATMENT FAILURE

It is now widely accepted that primary treatment of CIN should have a success rate of 90–95% for the majority of cases where the squamocolumnar junction (SCJ) is visible. This high figure would not apply to CIN where a cone biopsy was required because of disease extending into the canal. Under these circumstances it is difficult to ensure adequate excision at the endocervical margin. Risk factors for treatment failure include: large lesions; CIN3; older patients; and incomplete excision.

The term 'treatment failure' is intended to cover both residual disease, resulting from inadequate ablation or incomplete excision, and recurring disease. At which time-point we can strictly distinguish between residual disease and disease recurrence is a moot point. Disease that is identified 2 years or more following treatment, with normal cytology between times, is likely to be recurrence. In most cases a second lesion will have resulted from progressive enlargement of a residual focus, but in a few cases this will be a true re-occurrence, i.e. a new second lesion in the regenerated transformation zone. Treated women are generally thought to have an increased risk of developing a new lesion, compared with the general population. We know that the risk remains for up to 8 years, and therefore continued cytological screening is essential.

LENGTH OF FOLLOW-UP

Some insight into the pattern of treatment failure can be gained from a large study carried out in Aberdeen. A 94% success rate was identified following over 2000 laser ablations for CIN. Out of the 119 treatment failures, 70% were identified within the first 12 months, 24% in the second 12 months, and only 6% thereafter. This pattern probably reflects the three categories of treatment failure described previously. Follow-up during the first 12 months will generally identify truly residual disease. The second 12 months will largely identify very small residual foci that have enlarged and become detectable and the very small number of cases identified thereafter may well be true new lesions. This pattern of recurrence indicates the need for a more intensive period of follow-up during the first 12 months followed by a second phase of less intensive follow-up prior to returning to normal screening. Protocols vary, but a typical regime would be two checks in the first year, annual checks until 5 years, and return to routine screening thereafter. A recent intergroup study from four UK centres suggested that 10-year follow-up would be preferable because of the continued risk of post-treatment invasive disease.

METHOD OF FOLLOW-UP

The next consideration is the role that colposcopy has in the follow-up of treated patients. Cytology is the mainstay, with the need for colposcopy being more debatable. The obvious advantage of colposcopy is that of a safety net in the event of a false-negative smear, which can occur partly because residual lesions may be very small. One of the problems of colposcopy following treatment is that regenerating epithelium can sometimes resemble cervical intraepithelial neoplasia (CIN), because a rather prominent vascular pattern may be seen in the new transformation zone (TZ). In the previously mentioned follow-up study from Aberdeen, 20% of residual lesions were identified colposcopically in the presence of normal cytology. These lesions would probably have been detected cytologically over time, but early diagnosis has the advantage of identifying the need for a second treatment prior to discharge from the colposcopy clinic. A follow-up study from Newcastle has suggested that cytology is perfectly adequate for follow-up. The national guidelines accept that while colposcopy is optional for follow-up it may improve early diagnosis. In a recently performed survey of colposcopy practice in the UK, the majority of clinics reported the use of both colposcopy and cytology on at least one occasion.

FOLLOW-UP ROUTINES

A typical follow-up protocol would be as follows:

1. First post-treatment assessment: colposcopy clinic at 6 months, for cytology and colposcopy if the prior excision margin was incomplete.
2. Primary care (general practice): annually from 12 months to 5 years; cytology.

Thereafter the women would return to routine recall.

Following treatment, the SCJ usually remains visible, but on occasion it remains well up the canal (especially after cone biopsy) and thereby renders colposcopy unsatisfactory and of little value. Under these circumstances many will employ endocervical cytology with an instrument such as a cytobrush. If this is to be employed, it is better to use the colposcope first, because the endocervical brush usually causes bleeding, and this may obscure the colposcopist's view of the ectocervix.

In the future, human papillomavirus (HPV) testing may prove a valuable adjunct to follow-up, as HPV-positive tests confer an increased relative risk for detecting CIN within 2 years.

THE PROBLEM OF DEFAULT

One important practical difficulty of follow-up is that of the women who default. These women are at increased risk of eventually developing cancer, and a protocol must be in place to ensure that continued efforts are made to follow-up. If the patient defaults once, a reminder should be sent. However, if she persists in defaulting the best approach is to try to ensure that follow-up smears are taken by the general practitioner. It may be that the patient has moved away, or no longer wishes to attend the colposcopy clinic. Either way, communication with the general practitioner is essential. It is important to stress the necessity of follow-up at the time that treatment is carried out.

INVASIVE CANCER FOLLOWING TREATMENT OF CIN

Invasive cancer is the ultimate form of treatment failure after a diagnosis of CIN. If it is detected within 12 months of treatment, it is likely that there was early cancer present at the time of treatment. Microinvasive disease may be missed by an inexpert colposcopist and incompletely ablated by conservative treatment. The cumulative risk of frankly invasive or microinvasive cancer following treatment of CIN is 1m 200 over 8 years. It is almost inevitable that the occasional very early invasive lesion will be inappropriately treated by conservative therapy, and this probably accounts for the majority of such cases. It is possible that the increasing use of excisional therapy will reduce the number of invasive cases, because the occasional colposcopically undiagnosed microinvasive lesion may well be identified histologically in a diathermy loop-excised specimen, thus ensuring appropriate treatment. When the incidence of invasive disease falls as a result of improved screening, those cases diagnosed after treatment assume increasing relative importance.

FOLLOW-UP AFTER HYSTERECTOMY

Normally, the 15–20% of women who undergo a hysterectomy for reasons unrelated to CIN are removed from the screening programme, but this arrangement is altered if CIN is involved. There are three situations where CIN needs to be considered.

1. In women who had treatment of CIN in the past and subsequently underwent a hysterectomy for an unrelated indication with no CIN present.
2. Where a hysterectomy is performed for an unrelated indication, but CIN is an incidental finding.
3. Where a hysterectomy is performed as the treatment for persistent CIN or abnormal smears.

In general, provided that the hysterectomy specimen in the scenario 1 does not contain CIN, no follow-up is required. In scenarios 2 and 3, when CIN is present in the hysterectomy specimen, the correct measure is to undertake colposcopy of the healed vault to ensure there is no residual intraepithelial neoplasia and, if none is present, to undertake follow-up cytology of the vault (see Chapter 14).

CLINICAL PROBLEMS FOLLOWING COLPOSCOPIC TREATMENT

In general, the treatment of CIN involves little morbidity, but at the first follow-up visit an enquiry should be made about any symptoms experienced. It is not uncommon for women to mention some discomfort and irregular bleeding for a few weeks following treatment, but this usually resolves with time. Occasionally dysmenorrhoea is experienced and cervical stenosis should be sought, this being said to occur in 1–2% of cases. On occasion, cervical stenosis is seen at colposcopy in the absence of significant symptoms (see Chapter 15).

FOLLOW-UP COLPOSCOPY AFTER FAILURE TO DIAGNOSE CIN

In cases of mild and moderate dyskaryosis, colposcopy may not reveal an obvious lesion. If this occurs with a normal repeat smear then it is reasonable to conclude that CIN is not present and to discharge the patient. If, however, the repeat smear is again abnormal, it is best to repeat colposcopy at a visit in 3–6 months. If the cytology continues to be abnormal in the absence of an obvious lesion, it is permissible to treat the cervix – preferably by excision. This will encourage a return to normal cytology. Yet another scenario is when a directed biopsy at the first visit shows no significant abnormality. The likely explanation for this is a misdirected biopsy, and a repeat colposcopy and biopsy is again advisable in 3 months.

LEARNING POINTS

- The objectives of follow-up are to detect any residual or recurrent disease.
- The success rate of treating CIN is between 90% and 95%.
- Large lesions, high-grade lesions, incomplete excision, older patients and difficulties at the time of treatment are all risk factors predictive of treatment failure.
- Most treatment failures are detected in the first 12 months following treatment.
- Recurrence is likely when abnormal cytology follows a prolonged period of cytologically negative follow-up after initial treatment (about 2 years).
- Follow-up is based on cytology; additional colposcopy may enhance the early diagnosis of small residual lesions.
- Invasive cancer occurs cumulatively in 5 per 1000 treated cases followed for 8 years.
- Patients with a current history of CIN treated by hysterectomy require vaginal vault cytology follow-up.

MCQs

For answers to Questions, see Appendix C.

32. **After local ablative or excisional treatment of CIN:**
    a. The risk of frank invasive cancer is greater than in 1000.
    b. Most residual disease will be recognized within 12 months.
    c. Colposcopy and cytology should be performed within 3 months.
    d. Recurrent disease is more likely than residual disease.
    e. A success rate of between 90% and 95% can be expected.

33. **Follow-up for treated CIN:**
    a. Includes colposcopy at 12 months in all women.
    b. Is more likely to be abnormal in women who have had high-grade lesions treated.
    c. Is based on colposcopy rather than cytology.
    d. May be normal despite the presence of residual disease.
    e. Requires an annual smear for 3 years.

34. **After a hysterectomy:**
    a. Women who have never had an abnormal smear require no further cytological surveillance.
    b. Colposcopy and cytology should be performed at 6 weeks.
    c. Colposcopy and cytology should be a part of follow-up if CIN is present.
    d. There is a risk of vaginal intraepithelial neoplasia (VaIN) in all patients.
    e. Lugol's iodine is more reliable in detecting residual CIN than acetic acid.

35. **In untreated patients with abnormal smears:**
    a. Colposcopy may be normal despite a moderately dyskaryotic smear.
    b. The preferred treatment for persistent dyskaryosis is ablation.
    c. Two consecutively negative smears are required prior to discharge back to routine recall.
    d. Random punch biopsies should be performed if colposcopy is normal.
    e. A normal punch biopsy means that the patient can be discharged to recall.

chapter 13

THE MANAGEMENT OF EARLY INVASION AND ADENOCARCINOMA-*IN-SITU*

F.G. Lawton

EARLY INVASION

Once the dysplastic process breaches the basement membrane, an invasive lesion occurs. The depth of this invasion is measured from the base of the epithelium (either surface or glandular) from which it originates (see Chapter 3). This is important because it provides data regarding the risk of extra-cervical disease – either parametrial or nodal.

Initially in 1947, Mestwerdt suggested a definition of 'microinvasion' as a cancer penetrating up to 5 mm into the cervical stroma, but tumour depths ranging from 1 to 9 mm have been proposed.

The most recent FIGO classification defines Stage Ia as 'invasive cancer identified only microscopically', the lesions being subdivided into:

- Ia_1: measured invasion of stroma no greater than 3 mm in depth and no wider than 7 mm.
- Ia_2: measured invasion of stroma 3–5 mm in depth and up to 7 mm width.

Lesions wider than 7 mm are included in Stage Ib, regardless of depth of invasion, as are all macroscopically apparent lesions.

Other parameters apart from depth and width of the invasive process have been used to define prognosis (and hence treatment). A tumour volume of <500 mm^3 has been used to define the upper limit of microinvasion, but few laboratories have the necessary expertise – and indeed time – to examine cervical specimens with such rigour.

The presence of tumour cells within adjacent capillary spaces in the cervical stroma, so-called lymph-vascular space involvement (LVSI) is also cited as an adverse prognostic factor, but the significance of this remains controversial – most importantly because the definition of what constitutes a lymph-vascular space lacks clarity.

The invasive pattern (confluency) has also been cited by some as a prognostic factor, but no consistent definition of this parameter has been applied either. Finally, the cell type and differentiation has been considered as a prognostic factor, but as yet this has not been shown to influence outcome in multivariate analyses. One can only conclude that it is the depth and/or volume that relate to the frequency of nodal disease. As yet, all other parameters have not been shown to have a direct influence on this, but they may influence the risk of local recurrence.

DIAGNOSIS AND TREATMENT

A pre-clinical malignant lesion will, almost by definition, present as an abnormal smear. Despite arguments to the contrary, the colposcopic appearances of a high-grade cervical intraepithelial neoplasia (CIN) lesion and microinvasion can be similar, although occult cancer rather than CIN may be suspected by the findings of a raised acetowhite area with an irregular contour over which atypical vessels, punctation or mosaicism are seen. If the lesion is within the canal, the cervix may appear colposcopically normal. Most often, a microinvasive lesion is only diagnosed as the result of histological examination of a cervical biopsy.

With a 'see-and-treat' policy of large loop excision of the transformation zone (LLETZ) at the first visit for women with moderate/severe dysplasia on smear, the depth of invasion of such lesions can be ascertained, although diathermy artefact at the edges of the specimen may mean that absolute (or reliable) measurement of depth is not possible. If the diagnosis is made on a cervical punch biopsy, the patient should undergo either LLETZ or cone biopsy (Figures 13.1 and 13.2). It may be argued with reference to the previous sentence that in this case cone biopsy is more appropriate, and in either case it could be recommended that the procedure should be carried out under general anaesthesia in order to ensure an adequate specimen depth/volume to confirm the diagnosis of microinvasion.

INVASION LESS THAN 1 mm

Patients with invasion of less than 1 mm – so-called 'early stromal invasion' – have essentially a zero chance of either parametrial or nodal disease.

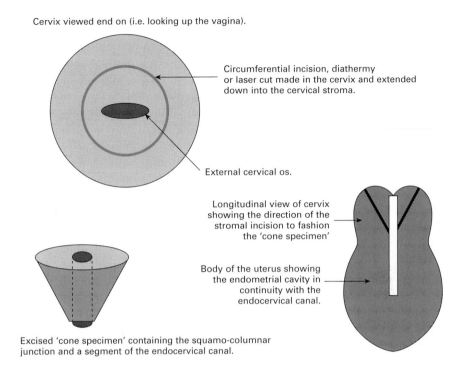

Cervix viewed end on (i.e. looking up the vagina).

Circumferential incision, diathermy or laser cut made in the cervix and extended down into the cervical stroma.

External cervical os.

Longitudinal view of cervix showing the direction of the stromal incision to fashion the 'cone specimen'

Body of the uterus showing the endometrial cavity in continuity with the endocervical canal.

Excised 'cone specimen' containing the squamo-columnar junction and a segment of the endocervical canal.

Figure 13.1 Diagrammatic representation of a cone biopsy of the cervix.

Consequently, provided that the histological margins are free from disease, curative surgery has already been accomplished by the LLETZ/cone procedure. Patients may opt for simple hysterectomy, particularly if fertility conservation is unimportant. Patients with positive LLETZ/cone margins should be offered simple hysterectomy or, less commonly, a second cone biopsy.

INVASION BETWEEN 1 mm AND 3 mm

Patients with microinvasion of between 1 and 3 mm have a less than 1% chance of nodal disease. The 3-mm limit may be associated with the width of the lymph-vascular spaces at this depth, their narrowness preventing the accommodation and hence dissemination of tumour cells. Cone biopsy is also adequate treatment for these patients if fertility is to be preserved: otherwise, simple hysterectomy should be performed. Oophorectomy is not necessary, as there is no evidence that these tumours are hormone-sensitive. There is no agreement as to the influence

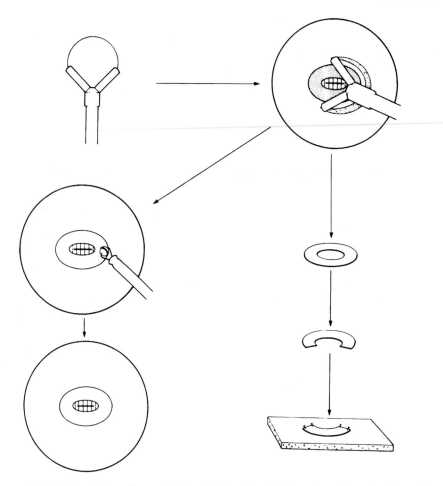

Figure 13.2 LLETZ excision of a small, fully visible ectocervical transformation zone. A medium (white) loop is used for the procedure.

of LVSI on prognosis in these patients, and controversy exists as to whether pelvic node dissection should be considered. One large retrospective study of over 450 cases of microinvasion did not report any improved outcome in patients who did undergo lymphadenectomy. The authors also reported a node positivity rate of less than 3% for cases with less than 3 mm invasion.

INVASION BETWEEN 3 mm AND 5 mm

The risk of pelvic node metastases in these patients is 5–8%, and here some authors have advocated a more aggressive treatment approach – particularly in cases when the lesion is greater than 1 cm in diameter, or more than 500 mm^3 in volume, or in the presence of LVSI. The recommended surgery, therefore, is a 'modified (or 'type II') hysterectomy', which excises the medial portion of the cardinal ligaments and the uterosacral ligaments, plus pelvic lymphadenectomy. (The standard 'type III' radical hysterectomy removes most of the cardinal and uterosacral ligaments and the upper third of the vagina along with the pelvic nodes.)

LESS RADICAL (FERTILITY-SPARING) SURGERY

Data from randomized studies to assess how radical the surgery needs to be in these cases are lacking, but it should be emphasized that deaths from recurrent cervical cancer after conservative surgery for microinvasive disease are extremely rare. A 30-year experience from The Norwegian Radium Hospital has shown a 2% recurrence/mortality rate in patients treated within such protocols. Other data have shown that simple hysterectomy may be adequate in cases after incomplete excision of early stromal invasion. Since there is little chance of uterine isthmus involvement in these early cases, logically, the uterine corpus does not need to be removed, thus providing the possibility of retention of fertility without compromising cure. In 1994, Daniel Dargent in France described the first series of women treated by radical trachelectomy. This technique modifies the established radical vaginal hysterectomy to remove the cervix, upper vagina and parametrium as well as the pelvic nodes, thereby dealing appropriately with the invasive cancer (i.e. achieving negative histological margins) but preserving fertility.

RADICAL TRACHELECTOMY

A procedure where data regarding outcome – and, more importantly, the cure rate is unknown and possibly worse than that of established radical surgery – should only be undertaken in established gynaecological cancer centres and after thorough counselling of the patient and their partner. The pathology should be reviewed, and further examination under anaesthesia and computed tomography (CT) or magnetic resonance imaging (MRI) studies performed to determine the tumour extent and volume. Criteria for selection for such surgery include:

- a strong desire to preserve fertility;
- the tumour being essentially confined to the ectocervix; and
- the tumours being of 'small volume'.

Tumours up to FIGO Stage Ib can be treated in such a way. The technique includes a vaginal approach when up to about 2 cm of vaginal cuff distal to the cervix can be excised. The vesicovaginal space anteriorly and the Pouch of Douglas posteriorly are opened, as in a vaginal hysterectomy. The ureters are mobilized and displaced cranially, and the descending branches of the vaginal and uterine arteries (but not the uterine artery itself) are ligated. The uterosacral and cardinal ligaments are ligated and excised about 2 cm from the cervix in order to obtain an adequate parametrial specimen. The cervix is separated at the isthmus, and a cervical cerclage suture inserted at this point. The associated pelvic lymphadenectomy can be undertaken either by laparotomy or laparoscopically.

Worldwide, data from over 200 cases are available for scrutiny. Short-term cure rates appear equivalent to those from radical surgery, and the 'take-home baby rate' appears to be in the order of 25%. Spontaneous rupture of membranes and pre-term labour seem to be greater in these cases compared with the normal population. Some authors have expressed difficulty in achieving adequate cervical dilatation to evacuate retained products of conception in failed pregnancies because of the cervical cerclage. Limited experience with this procedure and its confinement (quite rightly) to only a few centres means that this procedure should not be seen as standard treatment for early cervical cancer. At present, its only indication is in a woman with small volume disease and who desires a further pregnancy.

ADENOCARCINOMA-*IN-SITU* (AIS)

Invasive cervical cancers, which contain a glandular component, comprise about 20% of all cases – a number that has increased four-fold in the last 25 years. Whilst AIS is believed to be the precursor lesion to adenocarcinoma, it should be realized that it is detected much less commonly than its malignant counterpart – a very different situation from equivalent squamous lesions.

AIS is a more difficult pathological entity to characterize compared with its squamous counterpart. The earliest atypical nuclear patterns are subtle and may be confused with microglandular hyperplasia, or even normal endocervical cells. In addition, once the gland has been invaded, penetration of the nearby basement membrane cannot be measured with accuracy and consistency. Thus, the lesion is either '*in-situ*' or 'invasive'. Currently, there is no consensus among pathologists for a standard definition of 'microinvasive' adenocarcinoma.

The majority of cases of AIS are identified in cervical punch or LLETZ/cone specimens, or at hysterectomy for other conditions. Abnormal glandular cells may be seen on cervical smears, in which situation endocervical curettage and/or ultrasound of the uterus may be indicated. Over 60% of cases of AIS occur in association with CIN or microinvasive squamous disease. Occasionally, distinct squamous and glandular elements are mixed together as an adenosquamous carcinoma-*in-situ*.

DIAGNOSIS AND MANAGEMENT

No formal screening test exists for AIS, and there are no diagnostic colposcopic appearances of these lesions. In addition, since the lesion may be within the endocervical canal, the role of a colposcopically directed biopsy is limited. Only a cone biopsy can accurately determine diagnosis and extent of disease, although controversy does exist as to whether the whole of the canal can be sampled at cone biopsy. Some authors consider that only hysterectomy can ensure complete removal of the canal, but data have shown that if at cone biopsy the margins are negative, then the subsequent hysterectomy specimen will also be negative. Data regarding LLETZ as a replacement for cone biopsy are few and based upon small observational series, but it is likely that the length of the specimen achieved by LLETZ, particularly under local anaesthesia, would preclude adequate sampling of the endocervical canal.

Follow-up is also problematical, as great care must be taken to sample the residual endocervical canal that may be considerably scarred. A cytobrush or curette may be used to gain access to the canal, but it should be emphasized that one study concluded that "since one cannot expect to be able to thoroughly assess the endocervix over time, conservative management is dangerous . . .". There have been reports of recurrent AIS within a year or so of cone biopsy, and also of deaths from invasive adenocarcinoma 16 years after hysterectomy for AIS.

LEARNING POINTS

- FIGO criteria that are used to define microinvasive cervical cancer include depth of invasion below the basement membrane and surface area.
- Controversial prognostic factors include tumour volume, confluency and lymph-vascular space involvement.
- With a depth of invasion of 1 mm or less, the chances of lymph node metastases is essentially zero, and a cone biopsy is a curative procedure.
- With 1–3 mm of invasion, nodal disease occurs in less than 2% of cases. If the woman wishes to conserve her uterus (after appropriate counselling), then cone biopsy can be regarded as curative.

- The chance of lymph node disease when invasion is between 3 and 5 mm is 5–8%.
- The incidence of adenocarcinoma of the cervix has increased over the past two decades.
- There is no current consensus on a pathological definition of microinvasive adenocarcinoma.
- Cone biopsy may be considered curative for adenocarcinoma-*in-situ*, but a lesion high in the endocervical canal may be missed by such a procedure.

CLINICAL CASE SCENARIO 4

A 39-year-old woman, para 2+1, attended for colposcopy after a moderately dyskaryotic smear. Colposcopy revealed an acetowhite area on the posterior cervical lip which was considered to be CIN2, and LLETZ was carried out. Histology revealed squamous carcinoma-*in-situ* and also an adenocarcinoma-*in-situ*. The ectocervical margin was normal, but there were adenocarcinoma cells at the endocervical margin.

Questions

1. How should this patient's management proceed?
2. The upper margin of the specimen was positive and a further cervical specimen was required; this confirmed AIS, with negative margins. Six months later the cervix was colposcopically normal and a smear was taken that showed normal squamous cells only, with no metaplastic or endocervical cells. How should her management proceed?
3. In this case, the endocervical canal has not been sampled and the patient should be recalled. How can this be best achieved?
4. How can the endocervical canal be evaluated, given that unfortunately the cytology is still unsatisfactory?

MCQs

For answers to Questions, see Appendix C.

36. **Early, invasive squamous cell carcinoma of the cervix may be defined as:**
    a. A lesion with a volume of <300 mm^3.
    b. A lesion invading up to 5 mm into the basement membrane.

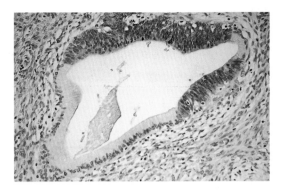

Plate 1 Gland showing classical adenocarcinoma-*in-situ* with an abrupt transition from well-ordered single-layer glandular epithelium to crowding and loss of nuclear polarity.

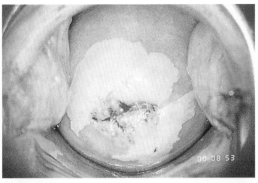

Plate 2 The atypical transformation zone: an extreme example of acetowhite change.

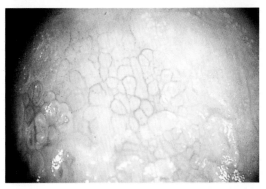

Plate 3 The atypical transformation zone: mosaic vascular pattern.

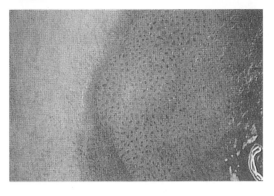

Plate 4 The atypical transformation zone: punctation.

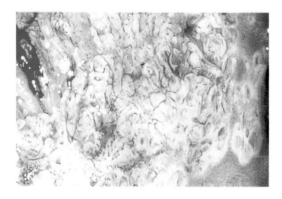

Plate 5 The atypical transformation zone: highly atypical vessels.

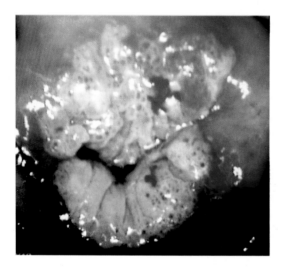

Plate 6 Early stromal invasion: coarse vascular pattern.

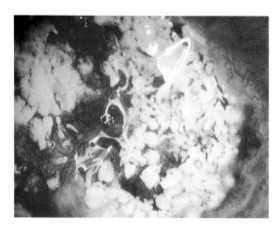

Plate 7 Microinvasion: dense acetowhite with coarse punctation and wide intercapillary distance.

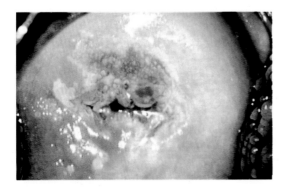

Plate 8 Microinvasion: irregular surface, dense acetowhite with coarse vessels.

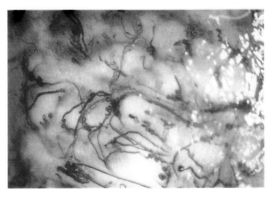

Plate 9 Invasion: abnormal vasculature – 'corkscrew' and 'comma'.

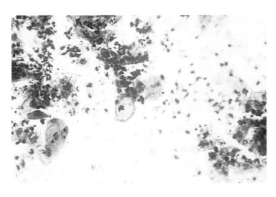

Plate 10 Inflammatory cervical cytology: background leukocytes may obscure and hinder correct interpretation. There are minimal nuclear changes.

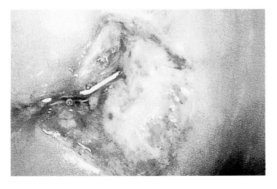

Plate 11 Primary syphilis of the cervix: the chancre would probably be misdiagnosed as squamous carcinoma at colposcopy. It is vegetative and friable, but possesses no typical characteristics.

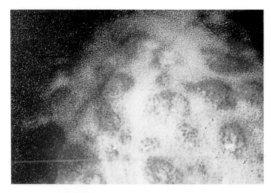

Plate 12 'Strawberry patches' of *Trichomonas vaginalis*: high power. This condition may be misdiagnosed by cytology or by typical symptomatology. The cervix often bleeds to the touch. Epithelial capillaries appear as clusters of red spots or 'strawberry patches'.

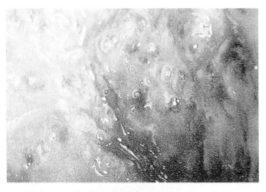

Plate 13 'Strawberry patches' of *Trichomonas vaginalis*: as seen with the naked eye.

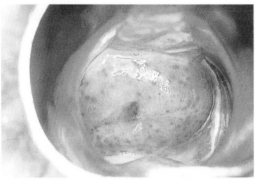

Plate 14 Herpes simplex: high power. Colposcopy shows vesicles, inflammation and ulceration of the cervix. Cytology may show typical 'foam cells'.

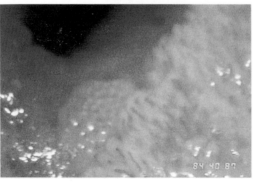

Plate 15 Human papillomavirus (HPV): high power. Colposcopy shows raspberry-like 'asperities'.

c. A lesion on the cervix which is invisible to the naked eye.

d. A lesion 2 mm deep and 8 mm wide.

37. **Fertility-sparing surgery may be considered in:**
    a. Stage Ia cervical cancer.
    b. Stage Ib cervical cancer.
    c. Adenocarcinoma-*in-situ*.
    d. A patient with a recurrent severely dyskaryotic smear after LLETZ for CIN3.

38. **Adenocarcinoma of the cervix:**
    a. Is decreasing in incidence.
    b. Has a defined microinvasive precursor lesion.
    c. Has a defined '*in-situ*' precursor lesion.
    d. Is found in nearly all cases in conjunction with an invasive squamous lesion.

39. **FIGO criteria used to define microinvasive squamous cell carcinoma include:**
    a. Depth of invasion.
    b. Tumour volume.
    c. Tumour area.
    d. The colposcopic appearance of the lesion.

40. **Radical trachelectomy:**
    a. Is associated with a poorer long-term outcome than radical hysterectomy.
    b. Should only be considered in women with no children.
    c. Includes bilateral uterine artery ligation.
    d. Does not allow such a large vaginal cuff to be removed.

chapter 14

HUMAN PAPILLOMAVIRUS: ITS ROLE IN AETIOLOGY AND SCREENING

G.P. Downey

INTRODUCTION

Cytological screening has been successful in lowering the incidence of cervical cancer. Although the test is specific for cervical intraepithelial neoplasia (CIN), and there is a low false-positive rate, there is a recognized deficiency in sensitivity. Given today's climate of high public expectation, it is unacceptable that up to 30% of tests are falsely negative (range 6 to 30%), and 30% of cervical cancers are associated with a (apparently) normal cervical smear within 3 years of diagnosis. In addition, between 16 and 30% of women with a mildly dyskaryotic smear have in fact high-grade cervical disease on colposcopy and biopsy. The ideal management of such women is immediate referral to colposcopy. Such a strategy would overwhelm an already taxed colposcopy service, and inevitably lead to overtreatment of some women combined with a major escalation in operating costs, despite many CIN lesions resolving spontaneously. These factors have led to a search for:

- a reliable alternative or secondary screening procedure; and/or
- a method of predicting which lesions would resolve spontaneously, and which would persist or progress.

HUMAN PAPILLOMAVIRUS

The importance of human papillomavirus (HPV) in the aetiology of CIN and cervical cancer was first proposed by zur Hausen in 1984. Since then, a wealth

Table 14.1 Human papillomavirus (HPV) subtypes in relation to oncogenic risk

Low-risk	**6**	**11**	42	43	44						
High-risk	**16**	**18**	31	33	35	39	45	51	52	56	58

Bold numbers indicate the most important in the UK.

of epidemiological and compelling scientific evidence has been produced to substantiate this claim. It is virtually certain that specific HPV types are the main cause of most cases of CIN and cervical cancer. Once this concept is accepted, then study of the viral structure, function, natural history and immunology can be employed to help manage CIN and prevent cervical cancer.

One of the problems of ascribing the virus an aetiological role in the development of CIN is its high prevalence in the normal population. Approximately 10–20% of all women will test positive for oncogenic HPV DNA, whilst 85–90% of women with a high-grade lesion will test positive, despite only a small proportion of them ever developing cervical cancer. The challenge is to predict who will progress – and why.

The different viral types found in the lower genital tract can be categorized by the associated risk that they confer on patients with regard to the development of high-grade or invasive lesions. By far the most important high-risk type in the UK is HPV 16, which accounts for 60–85% of high-grade CIN and cervical cancer, with HPV types 18, 31, 33 and 35 accounting for most of the remainder. The virus is transmitted by sexual intercourse, with infection often being transient and causing mild, reversible cytological changes. In a minority of women the infection persists and results in cervical disease (Table 14.1).

HPV STRUCTURE

The viruses are a family of double-stranded DNA viruses. The viral genome is divided into functional gene regions referred to as 'early' (E) and 'late' (L). The early regions contain eight open reading frames (ORFs) that code proteins concerned with viral maintenance and replication, while the two late region ORFs produce proteins that form the viral capsid and are termed 'structural proteins'. The latter appear to be important in the immune response to HPV infection. Although there is interest in vaccine development, little is known about which women should be vaccinated, and when. Vaccines, both therapeutic and prophylactic, currently have only a minor role to play.

Transfection of human keratinocytes with HPV causes cellular transformation that results in changes to a less-differentiated cell type. Integration of the virus into host cell DNA occurs when the cells progress to a more oncogenic phenotype, with each cell division typical of cervical intraepithelial neoplasia cells. Viral integration appears to play an important role in the oncogenic process, as the genes that control cell growth remain intact following integration while other viral genes are lost. Immortalization subsequently occurs in which the cell continues to divide *ad infinitum* rather than undergo programmed cell death (apoptosis) at around 40 cell divisions.

DIAGNOSIS OF HPV

HPV is tropic for the epithelium, and will only replicate in terminally differentiated keratinocytes; hence, there is no culture medium available for analysis. Serological tests are unreliable, and detection therefore depends on DNA hybridization techniques. Probes for the detection of HPV have been available since the early 1980s, and from a research perspective this molecular technology has yielded enormous benefits.

Southern blotting was regarded as the 'gold standard' test for identifying HPV infection, but whilst this test can be highly sensitive and specific it requires a large amount of DNA, is time-consuming and shows a loss in sensitivity when applied to cervical cytology specimens. Consequently, Southern blotting is not suitable for mass screening.

The **polymerase chain reaction** (PCR) allows for the enzymatic synthesis of millions of copies of a segment of target DNA. This technique is exquisitely sensitive and as such is now taken as the new 'gold standard', though because of its very high sensitivity and vulnerability to contamination it is not useful in mass screening.

Hybrid capture is one of the oldest nucleic acid hybridization techniques. More recently, a commercial form has become available which has refined the technique to be more sensitive and specific, yet still simple to perform. Initial trials reveal a high sensitivity and specificity for all clinically relevant HPV infection, and this is believed to be the technique of choice for mass screening.

SCREENING

The problem that faced proponents of HPV infection as being the 'cause' of cervical cancer was the relatively high prevalence of infection in the normal population. Because the prevalence of HPV infection is high, a simple dichotomous test that shows the presence or absence of HPV infection would necessarily have limitations. The inclusion of a quantitative test may allow greater sensitivity of the screening programme and rationalize management. Most data pertain to physician-collected samples, although recent data suggest that self-collected samples using vaginal tampons are almost as sensitive, thereby raising the issue of its use in underdeveloped countries.

HPV SCREENING IN THE PRIMARY SETTING

In initial studies the value of HPV 16 only was assessed to determine if it was useful to detect high-grade disease in an asymptomatic general practice population. The prevalence of infection in the normal population was high (16%), and the HPV 16 assay – assessed in a qualitative manner – was no better than cervical cytology in the detection of cervical disease. However, a combination of the two was better than either cytology or colposcopy alone. Similar studies have reported similar results, with an overall false-positive prediction of HPV testing in the region of 11%.

More recently, HPV types 18, 31 and 33 have been included in a study involving almost 2000 asymptomatic women with no previous history of cervical disease. The combination of HPV testing with cervical cytology was useful in the detection of those women with CIN, and had a greater sensitivity than either test alone. A much larger multi-centre study is currently underway in which HPV testing is carried out alongside routine cervical screening. The purpose of this large study is to determine the true usefulness of HPV testing within the context of the National Health Service cervical screening programme. The results are due for publication in late 2001.

HPV SCREENING AND MILD DYSKARYOSIS

By far the greatest problem facing the clinician is the 250 000 women with a mildly dyskaryotic smear report. As there is a recognized undercall rate of up to 30%, early referral to colposcopy would be the ideal management. However, resources are limited and this ideal is not practicable. The effect of the introduction of a semiquantitative PCR assay attempting to determine which women with a mildly dyskaryotic smear report have in fact high-grade disease has been formally assessed. HPV 16 alone was no better than cervical cytology, but a combination of the two improved the sensitivity of screening, without diminishing the specificity. A strong association was found in all these studies with medium/high copy numbers of HPV 16 (high viral load) and high-grade cervical disease, irrespective of the degree of dyskaryosis on cytology. Once again, the introduction of other HPV (types 18, 31, 33 and 35) has improved the detection rate of CIN3 to 84%. Other studies have confirmed these findings. The high sensitivity of HPV testing is critical with the predictive value of a negative result being extremely robust.

HPV SCREENING IN MODERATE TO SEVERE DYSKARYOSIS

Patients who have moderate to severely dyskaryotic smears will be referred for colposcopy, regardless of their HPV status, as these cytological results are much more sensitive and specific for high-grade disease than minor cytological abnormalities. Cytological screening for carcinoma and current high-grade disease remains more specific than HPV testing alone, and so the introduction of a HPV test would not influence the rate of referral for colposcopy.

HPV POSITIVITY AND FUTURE CERVICAL DISEASE

Natural history studies of HPV infection have been introduced in order to determine factors that influence HPV positivity, disease development and progression. It remains clear that environmental factors are influential, cigarette smoking in particular. HPV 16 seems to be the most predictive type for CIN of any grade. Because of this strong association of HPV 16, and the observation that low-grade disease that is positive for HPV 16 is more likely to progress to high-grade disease, research efforts to identify women at high risk of developing cervical cancer have focused on HPV 16.

Viral load appears to be an important factor determining an individual's risk for CIN development. In a recently published study in *The Lancet*, HPV 16 DNA-positive women with a high viral load were 60 times more likely to develop CIN than women who had low viral load or were negative for HPV 16. The HPV positivity predated CIN development by many years. Moreover, viral load appeared to increase in parallel with increasing dysplasia. In addition to high viral load, those women with persistence of HPV were at greater risk, this being especially true for women aged less than 25 years, 25% of whom will develop CIN. The time-frame from acquisition of the virus, high viral load and development of high-grade disease has yet to be determined. In addition, the exact level for 'high viral load' that defines high risk is also unknown.

LEARNING POINTS

- The present cervical screening programme has recognized deficiencies in sensitivity, with false-negative results and undercall of high-grade lesions.

Secondary screening measures using HPV tests, which are sensitive, specific, acceptable to the patient and cost-effective, have been proposed.

- HPV is a DNA virus that is sexually transmitted to the lower genital tract. Its natural history closely mimics that of CIN. There is a wealth of epidemiological evidence supporting an aetiological role for the virus in both CIN and cervical cancer. There are numerous viral subtypes, the main high-risk types being 16 and 18, with 31 and 33 playing an important minor role.
- There is no effective culture medium available for HPV, and detection relies on hybridization techniques. Hybrid capture is the most reliable and sensitive technique to use in the detection of all clinically relevant HPV infection.
- HPV assay alone is inadequate for the reliable detection of high-grade cervical disease. However, a combination of assays for HPV 16, 18, 31 and 33, assessed in a semiquantitative manner with conventional cervical cytology, can improve the detection of high-grade disease. Using this combined strategy may help to rationalize colposcopy resources and target referral to those who most require colposcopic assessment.
- Viral load and persistence of infection are important predictors of high-grade disease development.

MCQs

For answers to Questions, see Appendix C.

41. Regarding HPV and CIN, are the following statements true or false?
  a. The prevalence of HPV infection in the normal female population is approximately 15%.
  b. Hybrid capture is useful in mass screening.
  c. Quantitative HPV testing is as sensitive as cytology in detecting high-grade cervical disease.
  d. Viral load is important in predicting future cervical disease.
  e. Vaccines currently have a role to play in CIN prevention.

chapter 15

DIFFICULT SITUATIONS AND MANAGEMENT PROBLEMS

D.M. Luesley

ABNORMAL SMEARS IN PREGNANCY

There are two ways in which pregnant women present with abnormal smears: (i) they may have a smear taken during the pregnancy; or (ii) they may have had an abnormal smear and become pregnant before investigation and or treatment. With regard to the former situation, there is really no justification to take an *ad hoc* smear during pregnancy, though in some cases this might be the only opportunity of taking a smear and perhaps be a justification. The quality of smears taken in pregnancy – and indeed the early puerperium (6 weeks) – is generally poorer, and the risk of false negatives is higher.

ABNORMAL SMEAR RECOGNIZED FOR THE FIRST TIME IN PREGNANCY

The recommendations for referral for colposcopy are the same in pregnancy as in the non-pregnant state. Current UK recommendations are that all smears reported as moderately dyskaryotic or worse should be examined by colposcopy. Lesser abnormalities should be examined with a repeat smear 6 months following the first abnormality, and should be referred if still abnormal. One might also consider the possibility of undercall or sampling error, both of which are likely to be increased in pregnancy as a result of poor-quality smears, and the much larger transformation zone (TZ) that is a characteristic of the pregnant cervix.

For these reasons – and of course the more highly charged emotional state that prevails in this situation – colposcopy for all but borderline changes is perhaps the best option. As more women enter the screening programme, the need for *ad hoc* pregnancy smears has declined, and therefore the number of abnormal smear cases identified in pregnancy is also less. This means that an immediate referral policy will not significantly alter the workload of the colposcopy service.

COLPOSCOPY IN PREGNANCY

The procedure is no different from that performed in the non-pregnant state. Much more reassurance is required, with emphasis on the fact that the procedure will not harm the fetus or cause miscarriage. The cervix changes as pregnancy advances, with colposcopy becoming progressively more difficult. Because of this, misinterpretation is possible even in experienced hands. Women rarely need colposcopy in the third trimester, perhaps the only exception being late booking and a clinically suspicious cervix.

The major changes that affect colposcopy are as follows:

- The cervix is larger.
- Access can be more difficult.
- The TZ is larger.
- There is more mucus, and it is more tenacious.
- There is much more metaplasia.
- The cervix is softer and much more vascular (biopsy may be more morbid and small biopsies may be more easily damaged).

It is essential to take time to visualize the whole TZ carefully as a small field of cervical intraepithelial neoplasia (CIN) may be present within much wider areas of metaplasia. While accurate grading of CIN is important, there is a tendency to overdiagnose in pregnancy, with this perhaps reflecting the increased vascularity of the cervix.

The woman will need a large cervical biopsy if there is any suspicion of an invasive process based on the smear or on colposcopy. This is the most reliable way of excluding invasion. Small targeted biopsies are not ideal to exclude invasion. As treatment of CIN is rarely (if ever) indicated during pregnancy, there is little justification for taking directed biopsies, the reasons being that:

- they are unreliable in the diagnosis of invasive disease;
- in pregnancy, there is more chance of an unsatisfactory sample; and
- in pregnancy, there is an increased risk of haemorrhage.

For these reasons, large biopsies are preferable and are only performed if colposcopy and/or cytology suggests the possibility of invasion. Our own clinic protocol incorporates these ideas in a relatively simple structure that allows for minimal intervention in women with pre-invasive disease, yet provides an early diagnosis of those with invasion.

ABNORMAL SMEARS IN PREGNANCY: A PROTOCOL FOR MANAGEMENT

Such a protocol would include the following stages:

- Any abnormal smear other than borderline
  - Colposcopy within 4 weeks.
- Colposcopy and cytology suggest no more than CIN1
  - Repeat assessment 3 months after delivery.
- Colposcopy and cytology suggest CIN2 or 3
  - Repeat assessment at end of second trimester.
- Colposcopy and or cytology suggest invasion
  - Wedge biopsy under general anaesthetic.

POST-PARTUM ASSESSMENTS

These do not differ from those in the normal non-pregnant population. Occasionally, the vagina and cervix appear relatively hypo-oestrogenic, particularly in breast-feeding mothers. If this significantly hinders colposcopy and cytology, a 6-week course of local oestrogen often improves matters.

ABNORMAL SMEAR PRIOR TO A PREGNANCY

Women who have had adequately treated CIN do not require any additional surveillance during pregnancy. If a follow-up smear is required, this should be deferred until at least 3 months following delivery. The only group who should be offered colposcopy are those who have not had a negative smear after treatment where there are grounds to suspect incomplete removal of CIN, i.e. after incomplete loop excision of large lesions.

Women who have an abnormal smear but have not yet been investigated are managed as for those whose first smear was taken during pregnancy.

Women who have had CIN1 (or less) diagnosed should be reassessed 3 months following delivery. Women who have had high-grade disease (CIN2 and CIN3) diagnosed should be reassessed 6 months following the diagnosis and only re-biopsied (large biopsy) if it is felt that there may have been progression to invasion. Standard approaches are used to treat high-grade disease 3 months post-partum.

There are no published data supporting the concept of more rapid progression of CIN to invasion in pregnancy.

POSTMENOPAUSAL SMEARS

Women aged over 65 years who have had regular and normal screening are at very little risk of developing cervical cancer, and consequently the screening programme stops at this age. However, cancer of the cervix is still prevalent in older women, and current practice is that screening is maintained well into the menopause.

Some recently published data from Aberdeen and Dundee have suggested that well-screened women who have not had an abnormal smear can discontinue screening at the age of 50 years. It is likely therefore that as the screening programme in England and Wales matures, there will be a cohort of women who may be eligible for discontinuing screening 15 years earlier than is currently the normal practice. This might have major cost-saving implications.

As a result of oestrogen loss, profound changes affect the genital tract, including the cervix. There is an overall shrinkage of the tissues, with an inversion of the cervix, and as a consequence the squamocolumnar junction (SCJ) may appear to recede up the endocervical canal. Along with these changes the epithelium becomes thinner and more easily traumatized, there is less glycogenation of squamous cells, and the pH of the vagina increases, thereby removing one level of vaginal defence. Smears from post-menopausal women therefore contain fewer cells and less mature squames, and are less likely to sample adequately the SCJ. In post-menopausal women there is a greater incidence of unsatisfactory smear reports. There would seem to be good theoretical grounds for providing oestrogen replacement in such women and then repeating the smear.

COLPOSCOPY IN THE MENOPAUSAL WOMAN

Colposcopy is also less reliable in menopausal women as it is more difficult to fully visualize the SCJ and more likely to traumatize the ectocervix. Biopsies, which should always include the SCJ, will nearly always require some type of conization. This is because the shrinkage and inversion of the cervix cause the SCJ to recede into the endocervical canal.

Major degrees of cytological abnormality in elderly women should always raise the possibility of invasive disease – usually cervical, but occasionally even endometrial cancer might present because of abnormalities on a smear. Such smear results must be thoroughly investigated, with early recourse to a large biopsy and endometrial assessment. As future fertility is not an issue in these women, fear of anatomical distortion of the residual cervix should not deter the clinician from acquiring large biopsies. The indications for colposcopy are the same as in the pre-menopausal state. There is however a greater need for assessment if cervical smears are repeatedly unsatisfactory. Just as cytology is more likely to be unsatisfactory, so too is colposcopy. Apart from an increased chance of not visualizing the SCJ, the atrophic appearances can result in unusual vessel patterns. Prior cytology can easily strip the thinned epithelium, leaving exposed stroma, and in this situation the colposcopist cannot be sure that the removed epithelium was normal. The reaction to iodine (Schiller's test) is often incomplete because of poor glycogenation, whilst that to acetic acid may be false-positive because of stripping.

In situations where the smear definitely confirms dyskaryosis, conization is required unless colposcopy is absolutely satisfactory. If the smear shows very minor or borderline changes, treatment with oestrogen (locally or parenterally) followed by repeat cytology and colposcopy after 3 months is the preferred course of action.

ABNORMAL VAGINAL VAULT SMEARS

Women who have had a hysterectomy with CIN present require vaginal vault smears for follow-up. Other hysterectomized women do not. *De novo* vaginal intraepithelial neoplasia (VaIN) is very uncommon, and its prevalence far too low to warrant a screening test. Very occasionally women will have an abnormal smear who have not previously had CIN, and in most of these the cause is human papillomavirus (HPV) alone.

The vast majority of women who have an abnormal vaginal vault smear will have a history of CIN. To keep the number of these cases to a minimum, all women undergoing hysterectomy should have an up-to-date cervical smear and colposcopy, if this is abnormal, before hysterectomy. Colposcopy serves two functions in this situation. First, it helps to exclude the presence of invasive disease, for which simple hysterectomy would be inappropriate. Second, the colposcopist can see if there is any vaginal extension of CIN. If there is evidence of vaginal extension, then the removal of an appropriate cuff of vaginal tissue at the time of hysterectomy (vaginal or abdominal) should ensure complete excision of any intraepithelial disease. A careful histopathological assessment of the vaginal margins will determine whether excision is complete. Excision status determines the follow-up strategy:

- **CIN is confirmed in the hysterectomy specimen and is completely excised.** In this situation, a repeat vault smear should be performed 6 and 18 months after the hysterectomy. Follow-up should be discontinued if both are negative.
- **CIN is confirmed and excision is either uncertain or incomplete.** Follow-up is as for any treated patient with CIN. Vault smears should be performed 6 and 12 months post-hysterectomy, and annually thereafter to 5 years. If all the follow-up smears are negative, then 3-yearly recalls are sufficient.
- **Any abnormal vault smear requires a colposcopic assessment.**

VAGINAL VAULT COLPOSCOPY

This is more difficult to perform than a standard colposcopy as first, there is no TZ, and second, scarring and distortion of the vault because of post-hysterectomy healing can make full visualization of the suture line difficult. This is particularly so at the angles where, depending upon the technique of vaginal vault closure employed, deep inaccessible pockets can form. If these are present it is important to try and evert them with the aid of a small skin hook.

If abnormal epithelium is present it shares the same appearances as intraepithelial neoplasia with an intact cervix such as punctomosaic vascular pattern and acetowhitening. Any atypical areas should be biopsied, though this is also more problematic. Areas isolated from the suture line can be biopsied in outpatients, but the standard punch biopsy forceps may be difficult to use or cause an excessive crush artefact, as there is no subepithelial stroma. Atypical areas at or on the vault scar pose an even more difficult problem as sequestration of intraepithelial disease beneath the suture line often occurs. Some have suggested leaving the vaginal vault open after hysterectomy in all cases of intraepithelial neoplasia, to reduce the chance of burying CIN. This method of closure seems theoretically sound, but has not been proven.

A long-handled Keyes punch should be used to cut a good biopsy from the non-scarred part of the vagina. A formal **knife excisional biopsy** is the best technique when the atypical epithelium involves the angles or suture line. If excisional biopsy confirms VaIN and complete excision, the patient is followed-up as for after total abdominal hysterectomy. If incomplete excision is confirmed, there is a tendency to observe those where the original and recurrent disease is low-grade, but to perform a formal upper vaginectomy in confirmed high-grade disease. This is because several small series on post-hysterectomy VaIN have suggested a relatively high prevalence of carcinoma.

An alternative to upper vaginectomy is **vaginal vault irradiation**. This can be difficult to administer, and also has the potential to result in sexual morbidity as well as making any subsequent interpretation of vaginal vault smears difficult.

Chemosurgery has also been reported. This technique employs local applications of 5-fluorouracil for several days before using diathermy to slough the vaginal epithelium.

CERVICAL STENOSIS

Stenosis is a term usually reserved for situations in which narrowing of a structure causes abnormal function. Stenosis of the endocervical canal can cause symptoms such as dysmenorrhoea, and might also result in problems with conceiving or labour.

Stenosis can also cause the SCJ to become hidden within the canal, the result being non-representative smears and unsatisfactory colposcopy. Treatment of CIN is one of the most common causes of cervical stenosis, which occurs in up to 20% of cases following formal cold knife conization, but usually in 2% or less of cases managed by local destruction or local excision. Cervical stenosis occurs most frequently in women who are amenorrhoeic after cervical surgery (i.e. menopausal women). Reducing the length of canal removed reduces the risk of stenosis.

Women who are symptomatic require treatment. Cervical dilatation and/or recanalization by laser can be attempted, but this usually only provides short-term relief. Many symptomatic women will eventually need a hysterectomy.

Treatment is not usually required in asymptomatic women unless:

- **High-grade disease was present and was incompletely excised.** In this situation there is no reliable method of follow-up. Older women or women who have completed their families should consider hysterectomy in this situation.
- **Pelvic examination suggests uterine enlargement.** The possibility of either a haematometra or a pyometra should be considered. There is an increased risk of endometrial pathology in these situations, and again satisfactory surveillance or investigation is not possible. Hysterectomy should be considered.
- **Either of these situations prevails, but hysterectomy is not an option.** The canal should be dilated or vaporized at least to allow endocervical and or endometrial tissue to be biopsied. Women should be counselled that such measures are usually temporary and that re-stenosis is possible. In selected cases, an endocervical stent can be placed after dilatation. This prolongs the time before which further dilatation is required and may allow enough time for conception, should this be desired.

INCOMPLETE EXCISION

The method most frequently used to treat CIN in the United Kingdom is diathermy loop excision, either by large loop excision of the transformation zone (LLETZ). Diathermy loop excision provides a sample for the pathologist not unlike a small knife cone biopsy, apart from the fact that the edges of the sample will invariably show some degree of thermal artefact. The same is true with laser excisional cone biopsies. It is not uncommon for the pathology report to mention excision status, both at the endocervical margin and at the ectocervical margin. A statement suggesting incomplete excision often leads to a certain degree of clinician anxiety. However, this need not prompt a further excisional procedure for the following reasons:

- Although the specimen may show involved margins, the procedure may have ablated epithelium well beyond the margins, thus effectively removing any residual CIN.
- The process of excision may result in a further degree of tissue necrosis adjacent to the excision margins, leading to destruction of remaining CIN.
- The inflammatory exudate that follows excision contains populations of lymphocytes and macrophages that themselves may target atypical epithelial cells.
- Whilst follow-up studies indicate that large lesions and incompletely excised lesions are associated with higher rates of persistence of CIN, the majority of cases where there is incomplete excision are not associated with residual disease. Follow-up cytology with or without colposcopy is a far more sensitive indicator of residual disease than is excision status.

For these reasons, incomplete excision *per se* is not an indication for repeated treatment, but is a powerful indication for vigilant follow-up. The author would advocate that in all cases where there is a report indicating incomplete excision, both colposcopy and cytology should be performed at 6 months. Moreover, in the case of high-grade disease this might be extended to a second double assessment at 12 months.

There are two exceptions to this rule:

1. An incomplete excision and a report indicating microinvasive disease. Technically, it is not possible to accurately substage Stage Ia disease unless the whole lesion is present in the removed specimen. This is patently not the case if incomplete excision has been reported. When this situation does arise

(which is relatively infrequent), the author recommends recourse to a further large biopsy.

2. A report of incompletely excised adenocarcinoma-*in-situ* or cervical glandular intraepithelial neoplasia (CGIN), though this is slightly more contentious. Again, the author recommends a large biopsy in this situation.

Large biopsy in these situations should ideally be a specimen free from the possibility of thermal artefact, as this could interfere with subsequent interpretation. This is certainly one indication for a cold knife cone biopsy. When childbearing is complete, hysterectomy might be considered, although in selected cases of Stage Ia$_2$ disease, particularly if there is evidence of lymphatic space involvement, pelvic node removal might also be contemplated.

If cytology or colposcopy indicate possible persistent CIN after a report of incomplete excision, then further excision should be performed. Ablative procedures are not appropriate in these circumstances.

LEARNING POINTS

- Pregnancy and the puerperium are not ideal times to take a cervical smear. The quality of the smear can be affected by the pregnant or puerperal state.
- There is no indication to treat CIN in pregnancy.
- The main reason for taking a biopsy in pregnancy is to exclude invasion. A large biopsy is required to achieve this reliably.
- The natural history of CIN is not believed to be affected by pregnancy.
- The physiological changes associated with the menopause make cytology and colposcopy more difficult.
- As invasive disease is more common in post-menopausal women, there should be early recourse to excisional biopsies such as a cone biopsy.
- Oestrogen replacement may be valuable in improving both cytology and colposcopy in post-menopausal women.
- Cone biopsy is the most common cause of cervical stenosis.
- Cervical stenosis can cause symptoms and make cytology and colposcopy unreliable.
- All women having a hysterectomy should have evidence of a recent cervical smear.
- All women with abnormal cervical smears should undergo colposcopy prior to hysterectomy.
- Incomplete excision does not necessarily require an immediate further biopsy unless the lesion is microinvasive or glandular.

MCQs

For answers to Questions, see Appendix C.

42. **During pregnancy:**
    a. CIN is less likely to progress to cancer.
    b. Atypical features in the TZ are more obvious.
    c. Treatment of CIN should be avoided.
    d. Directed punch biopsy is the preferred method of excluding invasion.
    e. Acetic acid should not be used.

43. **With regard to the menopause:**
    a. Hormone replacement therapy (HRT) may help to cause metaplasia.
    b. Local oestrogen may help to improve the quality of cytology.
    c. Schiller's test is of more value than in the pre-menopausal state.
    d. Cervical screening can now be discontinued.
    e. Taking a smear can result in inadequate colposcopy.

44. **A pathology report of incomplete excision:**
    a. Means that there is a greater risk of persistent disease.
    b. Means that further treatment is required.
    c. Can be managed by either laser or another suitable ablative technique.
    d. Requires a directed punch biopsy if microinvasion has been reported.
    e. Can be followed up by cytology in the community.

chapter 16

COLPOSCOPY IN THE SETTING OF A GENITOURINARY MEDICINE CLINIC

D.A. Hicks

INTRODUCTION

Although approximately 300 000 women are seen annually in the genitourinary medicine (GUM) clinics of the UK as new patients, cervical smears taken from these patients account for only 1.5% of the 4.4 million smears performed nationally each year.

Offering colposcopy to the patient in the same venue that her other sexual health services are delivered is an attractive proposition, and fits well with the modernization agenda of the NHS. GUM colposcopy clinics, however, are no different from colposcopy clinics performed elsewhere in their requirement to meet quality standards, and neither should the GUM colposcopist.

Confidentiality may be requested by the patient in respect of non-identification to the cytology screening laboratory and, whilst this wish must be respected, fail-safe and follow-up of patients who often do not provide complete details, or who may be itinerant, is paramount.

Approximately 10 000 new patients are seen each year in GUM colposcopy clinics, with the colposcope being used in some GUM clinics to visualize other parts of the male and female lower genital and anal tracts.

ARE GUM PATIENTS A HIGH-RISK GROUP FOR CERVICAL INTRAEPITHELIAL NEOPLASIA (CIN) AND/OR CERVICAL CANCER?

First, some of the suggested risk factors for squamous carcinoma of the cervix should be considered. These include:

- Early coital debut
- Multiple sexual partners
- Smoking
- Human papillomavirus (HPV)
- Immunosuppression/human immunodeficiency virus (HIV)
- Suggested infective agents:
  - Herpes simplex virus (HSV)
  - Epstein–Barr virus
  - *Trichomonas vaginalis*
  - *Chlamydia trachomatis*
- Lack of participation in the cytology screening system.

The female GUM population generally could be considered therefore to constitute a high-risk group, and consequently the concept of being able to identify such a population in order to target resources is highly attractive.

Most of these factors carry only a relatively weak association with risk however, and it is currently impossible to identify that population which, if targeted within the programme, would substantially alter its success.

It should also be remembered that the majority of women who attend GUM clinics are under the age of 25 years. This age group contributes less than 2% of all cases of invasive cervical carcinoma, and only 0.2% of the total deaths from this cause. Rather, it is women aged over 40 years who constitute 70% of new cases of invasive carcinoma, and 86% of the deaths.

Since, to be more accurate, it is a short time lapse between menarche and coital debut rather than absolute age at first sexual intercourse that confers risk, it is not appropriate to perform cervical cytology on teenage women simply because they have been sexually active for a particular number of years. Indeed, the incidence of cervical carcinoma among teenagers is only 2 per 1 million of the population.

Similarly, women with a history of genital HPV or HSV infection have not yet been shown to benefit from more regular screening than National Programme intervals. Even if we assume that viruses pose a risk for the subsequent development of squamous carcinoma, this may occur many years after the initial infection. The woman may therefore be possibly disadvantaged in experiencing 'smear fatigue' when her initial smears are normal, with the system having to bear the cost of the increased number of smears.

HPV typing may be a valuable adjunct to cervical cytology in the future. Although its place is yet to be determined, it may help to triage women with borderline smears and/or in follow-up after treatment. Any introduction to GUM clinics, where 20–25% of the workload relates to genital warts, must merit significant research and consideration, not least around psychosocial and economic considerations.

The greatest contribution to the screening system for GUM clinics must therefore be 'opportunistic' cervical cytology, whereby smears are performed in women who, perhaps because of the lack of a general practitioner or a fixed address, have not been recognized or invited by the computer call/recall system, as well as in those who have not had a cervical smear taken within the previous 5 years (the maximum time period recommended in nationally agreed guidelines).

INFECTIONS, CYTOLOGY AND COLPOSCOPY

It is possible that an 'inflammatory smear' report may indicate the presence of an infective process (Plate 10). Specific organisms which may be identified on cervical cytology include HPV, HSV, *Trichomonas vaginalis*, *Gardnerella vaginalis*, *Actinomyces* and possibly *Chlamydia trachomatis*. Cervical cytology, however, is not a screening tool for infection, nor a replacement for appropriate sexual history taking and microscopic/microbiological testing.

Likewise, sexually transmitted infections are not in themselves an indication for colposcopy, though they may be present when it is performed. The following text briefly describes their colposcopic characteristics, but the reader should refer to a good atlas of colposcopy for pictorial reference.

SYPHILIS

The cervix is the sole site of primary ulceration in only 5% of cases. The ulcer is usually solitary and often mistaken for squamous cell carcinoma, but genital herpes, chancroid, tuberculosis, lymphogranuloma venereum schistosoma and Behçet's disease should also be considered, as well as an (infected) injury or drug-induced eruption (Plate 11). The lesion may be vegetative, but possesses no typical characteristics.

TRICHOMONAS VAGINALIS

The cervix may be seen to bleed when touched. Colposcopic examination shows a background inflammatory picture, with small epithelial capillaries appearing as clusters of red spots (Plates 12 and 13). These are caused by loss of the superficial layers of the squamous epithelium, and can appear on the cervix and/or vagina, being described as the 'strawberry cervix'. A 'leopard-skin' appearance can occur after challenge with iodine. The organism is readily identified on cytology.

CANDIDA ALBICANS

Candida produces an intense inflammatory response, with the epithelium of the cervix and vagina thickening and becoming covered with a curdy, creamy white discharge. Plaques adherent to the epithelium may bleed when disturbed, but should wipe away with saline on a swab stick, rarely interfering with colposcopic examination.

On cytology, spores and hyphae usually differentiate between active infection and commensal carriage (hyphae alone).

HERPES SIMPLEX VIRUS

The cervix is rarely the sole site of ulceration. The diagnosis will usually be suggested by a typical history and clinical presentation of vulval ulceration. Cervical colposcopic changes may be evident in the form of vesicles and epithelial inflammation, which are caused by cellular infiltration just prior to ulceration (Plate 14). The small vesicles seen early in the infection do not last long, ulcerating and coalescing to produce the more usual appearance of a single, serpiginous herpetic ulcer.

A constellation of symptomatology, history, viral culture and appearance can avoid the use of cervical biopsy to exclude malignancy. 'Foam cells' on cytology are very specific. Spontaneous resolution without scarring is usual and this is hastened by appropriate antiviral therapy.

HUMAN PAPILLOMA VIRUS

The appearance colposcopically of exophytic condylomata is varied, but their appearance on the cervix or vagina only (i.e. without external genital lesions) is very unusual.

Before the application of acetic acid, condylomata are soft, poorly defined tumours that often resemble small raspberries in colour and form, though they may also be pink or white. They are composed of fine, finger-like projections, each with a central capillary, which tend to be obscured when the papillae whiten after the application of acetic acid (the so-called 'asperities') (Plate 15).

The presence of exophytic cervical warts is an indication for colposcopy in order to determine the presence or absence of lesions in other sites, any associated CIN or vaginal intraepithelial neoplasia (VaIN) and to differentiate from the rare condylomatous carcinoma, which is an invasive squamous cell carcinoma integrated with condylomata acuminata.

The appearance of subclinical HPV on the cervix is described in Chapter 14.

OTHER PATHOGENS

Endocervical mucopus and hypertrophic cervicitis are said to be associated with *Chlamydia trachomatis* infection, and some suggest a typical cytological appearance. Immature metaplasia can be found also, as it can with cytomegalovirus.

WOMEN WITH HUMAN IMMUNE DEFICIENCY VIRUS (HIV)

Invasive cervical cancer in the presence of HIV infection is one of the list of illnesses that define AIDS (acquired immune deficiency syndrome). Whether the only underlying mechanism for the association is immune depletion or not is, as yet, unclear. The higher prevalence of CIN in immunosuppressed women, such as those with renal transplants, supports the view that impaired immune competency facilitates oncogenesis. Women infected with HIV may be at higher risk of developing cervical cancer independently of HIV infection, because of other risk factors.

Despite the risk for HIV-positive women, however, deaths due to cervical cancer are rare, possibly because premature morbidity due to other manifestations of AIDS occurs before the onset of extensive cervical disease. Nonetheless, this picture is changing because of the effectiveness of antiretroviral therapy.

The management of such women must therefore be a compromise and an attempt to balance the increased risk of developing cervical neoplasia with the need to avoid as far as possible, adding to the psychological and physical trauma that such women experience from other effects of HIV.

Women who are HIV-positive should be offered initial cytological and colposcopic screening to identify CIN. In those women who are found to have abnormal smears or CIN, management may need to take into account any coexistent HIV-related pathology.

Annual cytology with early recourse to diagnostic colposcopy is recommended, particularly in the presence of clinical immunosuppression, HIV-related disease and/or a CD4 cell count of less than 200 per mm^3. Whilst regular colposcopic examination has been advocated, its benefits are not yet clear. Moreover, the patient must not be denied any treatment on the sole grounds of HIV positivity.

MANAGEMENT OF CIN IN GUM CLINICS

'In-house' treatment and/or colposcopy of CIN has a number of advantages, including:

- **Counselling.** A woman who is already a GUM patient will have her cytology explained to her, probably at a subsequent routine clinic visit by health workers she has already met. A face-to-face discussion and explanation of the need for colposcopy can be detailed. Indeed, this may extend to an introduction to the colposcopy situation and equipment to help allay fears.

- **Continuity of care.** Colposcopy and treatment can be performed in the same setting and by the same staff already known to the patient.

- **Confidentiality.** The advantages of restricting an individual's sensitive medical information to the least number of people and case-notes is obvious. It is not contradictory to note, however, that disclosure of personal details to the cytology call/recall computer and general practitioner can also be to the patient's advantage. The case for and against disclosure can be put to the woman, and appropriate counselling should result in the correct solution for that individual.

- **Shorter waiting times.** When patients are referred 'internally' only, colposcopy and treatment clinics are smaller and waiting times tend to be shorter. This is a definite encouragement to attend. Some clinics perform colposcopy, as results become known, during routine clinics.

- **Fail-safe and defaulter follow-up.** Some women fail to provide their correct personal details when they attend GUM clinics. Others express the wish for their results, including cervical cytology, to be kept from their general practitioner. Some women request that no form of written and/or telephone contact is made from the clinic. It can be seen from the above that there is a potential for breakdown in communication, failure to disclose information and difficulty with follow-up for some GUM colposcopy patients. This tends not to be the case, however, since the above limitations are true of everyday management of sexually transmitted infections (STIs) and, with the intervention of a health adviser, potential problems can be avoided. GUM clinics should have a fail-safe procedure that takes account of the above. This must include increased commitment where correct information or communication is lacking or denied. In reality, default rates from colposcopy clinics in GUM are usually lower than in standard gynaecological colposcopy practice, probably because of the familiarity with, and acceptance of, the above.

CIN TREATMENT IN GUM CLINICS: CONCLUSIONS

The treatment of CIN 'in house' recognizes the concept of continuation of care. The GUM physician must be trained in colposcopy and treatment methodologies, and a theoretical and practical knowledge of the diagnosis and management of other pelvic pathologies is invaluable. Likewise, gynaecologists will benefit from a basic understanding of the management of STIs and close collaboration with their GUM colleagues.

Local methods of treatment are associated with primary and secondary haemorrhage in a small number of cases, and a few patients will require hospital admission. Close collaboration with gynaecological colleagues, extending to common management protocols and interdisciplinary audit, are to be commended. Treatment should not be performed where the facilities for admission and resuscitation are not immediately available.

LEARNING POINTS

- STIs are not an indication for colposcopy, and cytology is not an infection screen. The presence of STIs may modify colposcopic appearances.
- An increased frequency for cervical screening is not supported for the female GUM population on the grounds of sexual behaviour, age or history of STI. Opportunistic screening is valuable, and GUM clinics are ideally placed to implement this.
- Diagnosis and treatment of CIN must be to high standards of quality, accuracy and safety wherever they may be performed. GUM colposcopists should be trained to recognize gynaecological diseases, and gynaecologists should be aware of STIs.
- HIV-positive women should have annual cytology performed where appropriate, but management and treatment must not be denied on grounds of seropositivity alone.
- Confidentiality may extend to the non-disclosure of patients' names and other details to the laboratory, GP, etc. The advantages and disadvantages for the woman should be discussed with her, and her wishes respected.

CLINICAL CASE SCENARIO 5

Emily is a 38-year-old African woman who is applying for asylum in this country. She is known to be HIV-positive, and has a CD4 cell count under 100, with a viral load of more than 400 000 copies per ml.

Adherence to her antiretroviral treatment is episodic, and in the past she has been treated for *Pneumocystis carinii* pneumonia and syphilis. Cervical cytology has been performed in the GUM department, where severe dyskaryosis was found and colposcopy performed. The colposcopic appearance was suggestive of high-grade CIN, and biopsies showed CIN3 with HPV; the squamocolumnar junction was not visible. Cone biopsy was advised.

Questions

1. Do smears from women attending GUM departments have a higher likelihood of any significant abnormality being found?
2. Do women with HIV have a higher incidence of cervical dysplasia?
3. Are women who are immunosuppressed at increased risk for acquiring HPV infection?
4. Is cone biopsy contraindicated in women such as this with significant immunosuppression and HIV seropositivity?

MCQs

For answers to Questions, see Appendix C.

45. **In viral infections of the cervix:**
    a. A wart virus infection reported on a cervical smear is an indication for colposcopy.
    b. Cervical cytology is highly specific in diagnosing HSV.
    c. Women with a past history of genital HSV should have annual cervical cytology.
    d. Warts on the cervix stain white with acetic acid.
    e. HPV 16 and 18 infection demonstrates an acetowhite response; HPV 6 and 11 do not.

46. **In sexually transmitted diseases:**
    a. The 'strawberry cervix' is suggestive of *Trichomonas vaginalis* infection.
    b. *Gardnerella vaginalis* causes irregular branching of subepithelial capillaries, giving a classical colposcopic appearance.
    c. The pathognomonic cytological indication of HSV is the 'foam cell'.
    d. Exophytic cervical warts are an indication for annual cervical cytology.
    e. Some 5% of deaths from squamous carcinoma of the cervix in the UK occur in HIV-positive women.

47. **With regard to HIV-positive women:**
    a. The prevalence of high-grade dysplasia in HIV-positive women is esti-mated to be between 20% and 50%.
    b. HIV-positive women are more often infected with HPV than HIV-nega-tive women.
    c. The prevalence of cervical dysplasia increases as immunosuppression advances.
    d. Dysplasia amongst HIV-positive women is four times more likely to progress than in HIV-negative women.
    e. The prevalence of dysplasia in HIV-positive women increases with higher viral load measurement, even if the CD4 cell count remains stable.

chapter 17

COUNSELLING PATIENTS

T. Freeman-Wang and P. Walker

INTRODUCTION

Interacting with the colposcopy services because of the identification of an abnormality on a cervical smear can be an exceedingly anxiety-provoking situation. Women have explained that the shock of hearing that they have had an abnormal result is compounded by a triple threat. They perceive a threat to their mortality because the word cancer has been used, a threat to their fertility because they assume treatment will adversely affect their reproductive potential and, finally, a challenge to their sexuality because cervical cancer itself is often referred to as 'a sexually transmitted disease'. It should be the aim of everyone involved in the cervical screening programme to adopt strategies to allay these anxieties.

Generally speaking, psychologists recognize two types of coping strategy in people involved in medical treatment. For one group, their anxiety is compounded by a lack of information; these patients are called 'monitors'. In the colposcopy situation, if these women are given information at all stages, often in considerable detail, many of their anxieties will be relieved. The other or opposite group are called 'blunters'. For these women, too much information – especially of a detailed and medically orientated type – will actually worsen their anxiety. In different societies and in different parts of society the relative proportions of these two groups will vary, but the provision of information at all stages of the screening and treatment cycle, adapted for local usage, is essential.

INFORMATION AT THE SCREENING SMEAR

In many ways, the best time to explain the real significance of an abnormal result is at the time the test itself is performed. It should be explained to the woman that whereas it is expected that nine times out of 10, her smear will be normal, as many as one in every 10 women will be recalled. This may be for a smear abnormality (about a 1 in 20 chance), or because it is technically unsatisfactory for reporting (about a 1 in 12 chance). The chance of a smear identifying invasive cancer in an asymptomatic woman is about 1 in 1000. Therefore, it is best to say to the woman that if she should receive a letter saying her smear result is unsatisfactory, the most likely scenario is that it simply needs to be repeated. This may be for technical reasons, or there could be a minor change that needs checking in 6 months or so. There is a slight possibility that the cervix needs a slightly closer look with a magnifying glass and there is almost no possibility that an abnormal result means cancer. These messages, stated at screening and reinforced if necessary by an information sheet, should help all women whom later receive an abnormal result letter. Of crucial importance is that everyone in the practice or clinic – doctor, nurse and receptionist – should understand these figures and the relative risks involved so that a consistent message is imparted.

INFORMATION ABOUT COLPOSCOPY

It has been demonstrated that the anxiety experienced by women sitting waiting for a colposcopy examination is higher than that measured in women in hospital the night before major gynaecological surgery. Much of the anxiety can be alleviated if the patient receives, with the details of her appointment, an information booklet explaining in simple terms what the procedure involves, and why it is being performed. In the early days of colposcopy, such booklets were prepared by well-intentioned support groups but often inadvertently worsened anxiety. The original booklets would contain on the same page a description of cryotherapy and a description of radical surgery and radiotherapy. It has been found that a simple booklet written in lay person's terms, not in too much detail, is much more effective. The most successful information booklets are those that are personalized to the individual clinic, with a photograph of the hospital or unit and, if possible, of current members of the nursing staff so that the patient will recognize a friendly face when she attends. These fact sheets must also contain a few words reinforcing the point that the condition is minor, suitable for local treatment, often as an outpatient, and carries little, if any, risk to potential fertility.

In the psychology studies performed, one important fact was recognized and was a little surprising to the clinicians. Whereas, of course, the anxiety of the woman waiting for colposcopy was to a certain degree related to the disease process, an equal quotient was an anxiety about the performance of the procedure itself. One booklet contains the following advice to women on this issue.

BEFORE THE EXAMINATION

You may find it helpful to bring a friend with you. The examination is carried out in a room in the outpatients' department. You will first meet a nurse who will take you in to see the gynaecologist. In the room, after talking to the gynaecologist, you'll be asked to go behind the curtains and undress from the waist downwards. Before the examination the nurse will help you position yourself on the couch and ensure that your legs are comfortable in the leg rests. The procedure will last 10–15 minutes, so shuffle around to make sure you are comfortable and can stay in that position for the length of the examination.

THE EXAMINATION

At the start of the examination the doctor will take a smear in the same way as your general practitioner. After this, the doctor will look at your cervix using the colposcope. This is not painful. No anaesthetic is needed, and you will be conscious throughout the whole examination. In order to see any abnormal area the doctor will apply some liquids. The first is dilute vinegar (this may sting a little). As a final check the doctor may apply a brown liquid (iodine). The doctor may want to take a very small sample of tissue in order to look at an area more carefully. This is a biopsy and may feel slightly painful.

AFTER THE EXAMINATION

First, get dressed. The doctor will usually be able to tell you what the problem is, if any. If there is a problem, this will be explained to you and if you need treatment what and when this should be done.

"WHAT CAN I DO TO MAKE THE EXAMINATION EASIER?"

Remember
One in 12 women have an abnormal smear, so it is far from being a rare problem. Colposcopy is a simple, quick and painless procedure.

On the couch
Make sure you are comfortable. Shuffle your bottom to the edge of the couch. Make sure your legs are comfortable on the leg rests before the examination starts.

How to feel less nervous

- Remember – the colposcopist and nurse want to make the examination as easy as possible for you, so feel free to talk to them. Ask any questions you want to, however silly they may seem.
- Take deep breaths. Focus on relaxing. As you breathe out, try and imagine the tension draining out of your body.
- People find different things helpful when dealing with difficult situations. Some people find it helpful to focus on what is happening during the examination. If you think it would be helpful for you, ask the doctor or nurse to tell you everything as it happens. Focus on the sensations that you are feeling at each stage of the examination.
- Other people find it helpful to distract themselves from what is happening during the examination. To do this, choose an enjoyable daydream. Describe everything in the daydream in great detail including all the sights, sounds and smells around you.
- If you have any questions or worries ask the clinic staff. They are there to help you.

(Reproduced from *Your Visit to the Royal Free Hospital Colposcopy Clinic*, published by the Patient Information Department of the Royal Free Hampstead NHS Trust, London.)

INFORMATION AT COLPOSCOPY

At the colposcopy visit, the practitioner will wish to explain, to all except the most vehement of blunters, the basic physiology of metaplasia and the natural history of cervical intraepithelial neoplasia (CIN), even if the patient is already well prepared with adequate information having been provided at the time of screening. Many colposcopists will employ diagrams, often using a basic template of the uterus, cervix and vagina. It has been found most effective to draw on the template in front of the patient at the time of the consultation, rather than to have a series of previously prepared sheets. **Terminology** is very important, and using lay terms wherever possible in this situation aids women's understanding: neck of the womb for cervix; soft and hard cells for endocervical and squamous cells; changing area for transformation zone, and so on. The opportunity must be taken to state again the positive aspects of having been identified at this extremely early stage, that the woman does not have cancer, her fertility will not be affected and her sexuality is in no way being challenged.

There is little doubt that most patients with CIN3 and CIN2 who are not pregnant will be advised to undergo treatment. As well as details about the treatment itself, which will be discussed below, it is important to stress that untreated, between 30% and 70% of women with CIN3 will progress to invasive cancer, whereas once treated less than 4 in 1000 will do so in a lifetime. Important though treatment being conducted reasonably soon is, it should be mentioned that the mean length of time for CIN3 to become invasive is about 7–8 years. This additional information, rather than encouraging delay, simply balances the medical imperative for treatment at a measured pace and will deflect worry that the patient thinks she may have (or is about to get) cancer itself.

As most will accept, the situation with regard to CIN1 is far less clear-cut. The patient will need to make her own decision on the evidence that only 14% of CIN1 lesions progress to CIN3, let alone cancer, whereas 86% will remain at the level of CIN1 or regress completely over 10 years. She will also need to balance the possibilities of the conservative approach against the disadvantage of non-treatment, which entails 6-monthly colposcopic visits, possibly for some years ahead. In this situation, it is the role of her doctor simply to provide her with accurate information and direct her decision-making only if requested so to do.

INFORMATION ABOUT TREATMENT

Information sheets about treatment were amongst the first patient fact sheets introduced in many colposcopy clinics. Certain key points should be covered (Figure 17.1). It is important to stress that the treatment is minor, common up and down the country, and successful. Most would tell their patients about a 95% first-time treatment success rate with resort to further treatment for the minority, this usually involving a second simple treatment rather than anything more drastic. It should be stated that most treatments are performed under local anaesthesia, but that some women require and others may request a short, day-case general anaesthetic instead. Most importantly, information will be required about the possibility, type, nature and severity of bleeding postoperatively and this should be described in terms the woman can understand.

Most – but perhaps not all – would advise their patients not to use tampons, and to avoid penetrative vaginal intercourse for 4 weeks after treatment, and if this is the local advice it should be in the leaflet. It is vital that the fact sheet contains contact names and contact numbers which the patients can use if they are worried about an expected or unexpected side effect or symptom during the recovery period. There should ideally be a telephone line devoted to this use only, with additional information about what to do and who to contact out of hours

Dear . . . .

Laser/LLETZ treatment is a method of removing abnormal tissue from the cervix. In your particular case, this means taking away the abnormal area on the neck of the womb with a 95% chance of cure with just one treatment. Occasionally, a shorter second treatment may be required. Treatment can be carried out in the outpatients department with a local anaesthetic, or occasionally as an inpatient under general anaesthesia.

There is very little discomfort associated with the treatment; some experience a period-like pain, which goes away as soon as the treatment is completed.

Following laser/LLETZ treatment, one or two points must be observed:

1. Please DO NOT take any severe exercise for TEN DAYS.
2. For the first 4 weeks following treatment, DO NOT place anything in the vagina, i.e. no douching, no tampons, and do not have intercourse.

You may experience some bleeding following therapy. This may not start for a few days, and may last as long as 2 weeks. The bleeding may be anything from slight spotting to a flow as heavy as an average period. If the bleeding persists after 2 weeks, or is so heavy as to cause you to change a max-pad every 2 hours or more, or if you are worried in any way, then please ring 000000000 and a gynaecological sister will be able to advise you. Only three women in every hundred actually require any extra treatment because of heavy bleeding.

Laser/LLETZ therapy requires follow-up. You will be given an appointment for a simple check up for 6 weeks following treatment, and also an appointment for a repeat smear at 6 months after treatment. Following one further smear 6 months later, we hope that you will then simply have to attend for an annual cervical smear.

Happily, a single laser/LLETZ treatment has no adverse effect on future fertility, pregnancy or labour.

Figure 17.1 A typical patient information sheet.

and at weekends. Finally, the precise nature of the follow-up protocol should be described and the importance of follow-up stressed. Interestingly, it is quite easy to place all this information on one sheet of A4 paper.

INFORMATION ABOUT 'SEE-AND-TREAT'

In recent years, the majority of units in the UK have introduced 'see-and-treat' clinics. Whereas the traditional approach to treatment involved the woman attending the clinic on two occasions, the first visit for colposcopy and biopsy, the second for a subsequently arranged treatment appointment, 'see-and-treat' clinics have offered diagnosis and treatment at the first hospital attendance.

Initially, the introduction of such clinics resulted in the overtreatment of women with minor grade disease. Recently, the National Quality Assurance in Colposcopy group has recommended that women should only be managed in a 'see-and-treat' clinic under the following circumstances:

- They have been referred with a moderate or severely dyskaryotic smear.
- There is an identifiable lesion on the cervix.
- The woman has received adequate pre-visit information, allowing her to make an informed choice as to whether she wants to undergo treatment.

Although it has been recognized there are high levels of anxiety in women attending for colposcopy, little information has previously been available about anxiety levels at the time of treatment. A study at The Royal Free Hospital, London identified that whereas anxiety levels in women attending the traditional second visit for treatment were similar to those high levels in women attending their first visit, the levels measured in women attending a 'see-and-treat' clinic were significantly higher still. A randomized controlled trial in which one group of patients were given standard leaflet information, but the second group were given a specifically designed video, demonstrated that pre-visit video information could substantially reduce levels of anxiety to a point below even that experienced at first attendance.

The key elements of the video information were that it provided women with:

- Images of the unit itself and the staff who would look after the woman at her hospital attendance.
- A description of the pathophysiology of CIN and the rationale for treatment.
- A description of the treatment itself, possible side effects and complications and details of required aftercare.

Not all units would wish or would be able to introduce an in-house video. However, women attending 'see-and-treat' appointments must be identified as a potentially very anxious and vulnerable group who require additional information and counselling. Other approaches for these women might include more detailed written information, or the opportunity to meet a nurse counsellor prior to their visit.

COMMON PATIENT CONCERNS

However thorough the information sheets, and however talented as communicators the doctors and nurses might be, unfortunately many patients will be left with unanswered questions and they must be encouraged to articulate these.

SEX AND PROMISCUITY

There has been much – in fact, too much – attention paid in the medical and lay press to the possible sexually transmitted nature of cervical cancer and its precursors. As a result, many women feel embarrassed and worried about the implications of this. Reassurance can be given to one group in particular by stating that 15% of cervical cancer is a glandular condition which, as far as we know, has nothing whatever to do with sexual behaviour. Although squamous cancer only occurs in women who are or have been sexually active, it must be stressed that squamous cancer itself and CIN says nothing about a woman, her behaviour, her number of partners or their behaviour. For this reason such questions should never be asked of women at colposcopy, except and unless a clearly defined research study has been identified and approved. As far as the individual woman is concerned, her sexuality and behaviour are nothing to do with colposcopy or her colposcopist.

VIRUSES AND PARTNERS

It is now generally accepted that high-risk HPV types are necessary – if not sufficient – for the development for high-grade CIN and cervical cancer. It is probable that testing for these high-risk viral types will be introduced in some form into the National Health Service Cervical Screening Programme (NHSCSP) in the next few years. The introduction may involve testing for the viral types as a secondary screen for women with minor cytological abnormalities, or ultimately it may form part of the initial 3-yearly screening process.

As the introduction of these novel technologies evolves, women will request and require additional information and reassurance about the true significance of a positive HPV test. Women should be informed that genital HPV infections are common, with up to 70% of women testing positive for genital HPV in longitudinal studies. The majority of women clear HPV from their genital tract in an average time of 8 to 10 months. It is the smaller group of women in whom high-risk HPV types persist that significant CIN and the need for treatment may occur.

Although treatment for CIN is not strictly speaking anti-viral therapy, the majority of women treated for CIN will subsequently test negative for the virus.

Given the high prevalence of virus in the normal sexually active population, women can perhaps be reassured that anxieties about "When did I get the virus", "Who gave it to me" and "Can I give it to others?" are not questions the clinician can answer.

CONTRACEPTION AND PREGNANCY

There is no indication for a woman to be advised to change her method of contraception. There is no evidence of the specific need to recommend the use of barrier contraception in women with CIN, or those who have been treated for it.

FUTURE FERTILITY

There is no evidence that a single treatment for CIN by a locally destructive or non-knife-cone biopsy local excisional technique has any adverse effect on a woman's future fertility, pregnancy, carriage or delivery. It is to be hoped that the same will prove to be the case for those treated twice with these methods but, as yet, there are no data available.

CIN IN PREGNANCY (see also Chapter 15)

There is no reason to treat CIN in pregnancy, provided that an expert colposcopist has confirmed the pre-invasive nature of the lesion. There is no evidence that the CIN process is accelerated by pregnancy; the only delay that occurs is delay in treatment until after delivery. CIN is not affected by vaginal delivery, and CIN and even HPV (as far as we know) have absolutely no adverse effect on the fetus or baby.

These clear and simple messages should be reinforced for all women.

SUMMARY

Great care is required in counselling women about colposcopy and CIN. Information booklets personalized to the unit and expressed in simple terms, preferably with input in design from previous and current patients, can allay many of the anxieties women feel when they have an abnormal smear.

LEARNING POINTS

- Many women experience anxiety as a result of cervical screening and interaction with colposcopy services because the diagnosis of an abnormal smear presents potential threats to their sexuality, fertility and mortality.
- Much of the anxiety associated with the screening programme and colposcopy can be alleviated by providing patients with adequate information in written and in visual form, supported by verbal explanation at all points in the process.
- High-risk HPV types are necessary if not sufficient for the development of high-grade disease cervical cancer.
- The true natural history of viral-associated minor epithelial abnormalities of the cervix remains unclear.

MCQs

For answers to Questions, see Appendix C.

48. **When counselling women, are the following true or false?**
    a. Women waiting for a colposcopy examination are more anxious than those awaiting major surgery.
    b. A full sexual history should always be taken as part of a woman's colposcopy assessment.
    c. Detailed information booklets are most effective in reducing anxiety.
    d. A 'see-and-treat' policy is less anxiety-provoking than a 'select-and-treat' policy for women.
    e. The large majority of women with CIN1 left untreated would not develop cervical cancer.
    f. Simple written information specific to each colposcopy unit is as effective as video information.
    g. Up to 70% of women will test positive for genital HPV infection at some stage in their reproductive life.

chapter 18

EDUCATION, TRAINING AND ACCREDITATION IN COLPOSCOPY

C.W.E. Redman

INTRODUCTION

The outcome of colposcopy depends upon the skill and knowledge of the colposcopist, and the context or clinical setting in which it is applied. Being observer-dependent, colposcopic findings will always be somewhat subjective, whilst the subsequent decisions and patient management requires experience and problem-solving skills. Given these facts, it follows that achieving high standards in diagnosis and management requires not only an appropriate training but also an adequate caseload and casemix in order to maintain skills.

Throughout the developed world there are increasing concerns regarding quality and cost-effectiveness of healthcare services.

With regard to colposcopy, protection against substandard practice is particularly relevant given its subjective nature, the large numbers of patients involved, and the fact that most of these patients are fit and well. When performed well, colposcopy can minimize damage, but if performed badly then the scope for unnecessary morbidity is high. One must acknowledge that while the indications for colposcopy may vary throughout Europe, its objective remains the same – that is, the detection of asymptomatic precursor lesions of cervical cancer.

The above facts partly explain the priority given now by national and international groups to work toward standardization of colposcopic training and agreement over methods of audit.

In the United Kingdom, the British Society of Colposcopy and Cervical Pathology (BSCCP), along with the National Health Service Cervical Screening Programme (NHSCSP) and the Royal College, have begun to develop modular training programmes in tandem with quality control procedures. Although this represents the activities in only one country, there are useful lessons to be learned from this UK experience.

THE UNITED KINGDOM EXPERIENCE

In the UK, colposcopy is performed as part of the NHSCSP. Women aged between 20 and 65 years are invited to have a cervical smear on a three- to five-yearly basis; this serves as a primary screen to select patients for further colpo-scopic assessment. Using a computerized call and recall system, up to 93% of the targeted population – approximately 4 000 000 women – are screened each year, and of these about 100 000 are referred for colposcopy.

Cytological practice in the UK has been the subject of both internal and external quality control, and well-defined training criteria have been in place for some time. However, colposcopy has lagged behind somewhat, and only now has a more systematic training process been adopted along with a requirement for quality assurance.

In 1996, a working party involving the various parties involved in the screening programme recommended that there should be an agreed training programme. The BSCCP responded to these recommendations and launched an accreditation process. In conjunction with Royal College of Obstetricians and Gynaecologists (RCOG), a structured training programme was also introduced, which all future colposcopists will need to complete successfully in order to practice as BSCCP-certified colposcopists.

BSCCP CERTIFICATION FOR COLPOSCOPY

The NHSCSP colposcopy quality standards require that all colposcopists are adequately trained and also see sufficient patients to maintain their skills. The BSCCP has set the goal that all patients undergoing colposcopy are seen either by BSCCP-certified colposcopists, or by trainees under supervision. At present, certification occurs on a triennial basis and requires the colposcopist to:

- demonstrate a sufficient work-load, which is defined as a minimum of 50 new patients per annum;
- make a commitment to audit; and
- take part in continued medical education, i.e. they must attend at least one BSCCP-recognized meeting every 3 years.

THE BSCCP/RCOG TRAINING PROGRAMME

The programme is open to any qualified doctor or nurse who has attended a BSCCP-recognized Basic Colposcopy Course. The trainee must identify a trainer, who should be recognized by the BSCCP as a certified colposcopist. The trainee should then register his or her intent to train with the BSCCP. It has been estimated that the NHSCSP needs about 40 new colposcopists a year to maintain the current manpower status quo.

The training programme is trainee-centred and has an agreed structured curriculum. The trainee must see a total of 150 patients under supervision (the first 50 of these must be directly supervised, after which a formative assessment is carried out). The trainee is required to present 10 short case commentaries on which the management is discussed, this being in addition to completing a log-book. Successful completion of these requirements allows the trainee to be awarded the BSCCP/RCOG Colposcopy (D) diploma, i.e. in diagnostic colposcopy. There is an optional treatment module which allows the BSCCP/ RCOG Colposcopy (DT) diploma, i.e. diagnosis and treatment.

POSITIVE ASPECTS OF THE TRAINING PROGRAMME

The training programme and accreditation process evolved from basic principles that had as their basis avoidance of complexity and clear, achievable targets in an attempt to promote a degree of quality. It demonstrates what can be achieved when there is a clear vision and the involved professionals are allowed to introduce an initiative, without external interference.

In a relatively short space of time this system of accreditation and training has been comprehensively and successfully introduced from scratch. This has been a notable achievement. There are a number of factors that have facilitated this initiative. The majority of UK colposcopy is practised within the NHS, which has during this period been increasingly concerned with audit, clinical governance and quality. The NHS is responsible for virtually all medical and nursing training in the UK.

Colposcopy forms part of the NHSCSP, and this has helped to introduce a uniform strategy based on agreed quality standards. Through previously agreed national guidelines, the role of – and indications for – colposcopy have been well defined. There has been close co-operation between the NHSCSP and the involved national bodies, which include the BSCCP, RCOG, and the Association of Genito-Urinary Medicine. The BSCCP is a well-established and thriving society that has promoted colposcopy for over 25 years, and a society to which most UK colposcopists belong. All these factors have promoted consensus and cohesion.

PROBLEMS WITH THE PROGRAMME

At the outset, although there was an implied goal for the training programme, the formal educational goals were never formally identified. Although many accepted educational principles have been incorporated, the training programme has had no formal input in those with a predominant background in education. This has been partly addressed in a formal curriculum review which included consultation with stakeholders, e.g. the NHSCSP. Nonetheless, this is a training programme that has minimal quality control and no objective assessment of the product, namely the trained colposcopist.

The quality of a training programme is dependent on the trainers, and currently the only requirement to become a trainer is to be a BSCCP-certified colposcopist. Many trainers will not have received educational training, and consequently their abilities to train must vary. Apart from auditing some of the case commentaries (which may reflect the quality of training), there is no training quality assurance. Measures to address this shortcoming are being discussed, including seeking feed-back from trainees and considering the possibility of some form of 'exit' assessment – as occurs in other professional areas, such as in obstetric ultrasound. It must be said that colposcopy is not unique in this deficit, and many areas of medical education are likely to suffer from the same shortcomings.

The majority of UK colposcopists are now BSCCP-certified but, in isolation, this does not guarantee quality. Most certified colposcopists achieved accreditation via 'self-certification' whereby practising colposcopists trained before April 1998 were eligible for accreditation if, in addition to seeing adequate numbers and having a commitment to audit and continued medical education, they stated that their training had been adequate. Re-certification may enable some degree of quality assurance by requiring returns of activity, thereby enabling audit of their practice against nationally agreed quality standards. The first re-certification exercise has only just taken place, and the object is simply to complete a limited data form (this will allow an audit of a limited number of standards, though achieving these is not necessary for an individual to remain accredited). The ultimate objective is to link quality assurance of the service (which has just been introduced) with that of the individual colposcopist. This goal should be achievable using the common electronic dataset that is the basic tool of National QA.

WHAT HAVE WE LEARNED SO FAR?

In a relatively short space of time, a comprehensive accreditation and training programme has been instituted. In many ways the scene was set for this to happen, as throughout the NHS a quality assurance culture has emerged, responding to a political and public demand for cost-effectiveness and account-ability. There appeared to be a high degree of consensus that these changes were right and necessary, and consequently little opposition has been encountered.

Another factor that promoted the implementation of these initiatives was the uniformity of healthcare provision. Throughout the UK, colposcopy is a compo-nent part of the NHSCSP, and is usually undertaken as a secondary-screening test on cases selected by cervical cytology, according to national guidelines. The screening strategy and its prosecution involves relatively few agencies which have considerable influence on practice; once decisions are made they can be imple-mented relatively easily, illustrating the value of a recognized organizational structure.

The various changes introduced were kept simple with a view to increasing stringency and sophistication with time rather than bringing in wholesale a complicated package that would fail through impracticality.

APPENDIX A: FIGO STAGING OF CERVICAL CANCER

Stage I

The carcinoma is strictly confined to the cervix (extension to the corpus should be disregarded).

- *Stage Ia:* Invasive cancer identified only microscopically. All gross lesions, even with superficial invasion, are stage 1b cancers.

  Invasion is limited to measured stromal invasion with a maximum depth of 5 mm and no wider than 7 mm.*
  - Stage Ia_1: Measured invasion of stroma no greater than 3 mm in depth and no wider than 7 mm.
  - Stage Ia_2: Measured invasion of stroma greater than 3 mm and no greater than 5 mm in depth and no wider than 7 mm.
- *Stage Ib:* Clinical lesions confined to the cervix or pre-clinical lesions greater than Ia.
  - Stage Ib_1: Clinical lesions no greater than 4 cm in size.
  - Stage Ib_2: Clinical lesions greater than 4 cm in size.

Stage II

The carcinoma extends beyond the cervix, but has not extended on to the pelvic wall. The carcinoma involves the vagina, but not as far as the lower third.

- *Stage IIa:* No obvious parametrial involvement.
- *Stage IIb:* Obvious parametrial involvement.

Stage III

The carcinoma has extended on to the pelvic wall. On rectal examination there is no cancer-free space between the tumour and the pelvic wall.

The tumour involves the lower third of the vagina. All cases with a hydronephrosis or non-functioning kidney should be included, unless they are known to be due to other cause.

- *Stage IIIa:* No extension on to the pelvic wall, but involvement of the lower third of the vagina.
- *Stage IIIb:* Extension on to the pelvic wall or hydronephrosis or non-functioning kidney.

Stage IV
The carcinoma has extended beyond the true pelvis or has clinically involved the mucosa of the bladder or rectum.

- *Stage IVa:* Spread of the growth to adjacent organs.
- *Stage IVb:* Spread to distant organs.

*Note: The depth of invasion should not be more than 5 mm taken from the base of the epithelium, either surface or glandular, from which it originates. Vascular space involvement, whether venous or lymphatic, should not alter the staging.

APPENDIX B: COLPOSCOPIC TERMINOLOGY AND TECHNIQUE

TERMINOLOGY

HISTOLOGICAL TERMS

- **Original squamous epithelium** is the squamous epithelium that is laid down at the time of organogenesis. Usually, it covers the vagina and most of the ectocervix.
- **Original columnar epithelium** refers to columnar epithelium laid down at the time of organogenesis. It is usually confined to the endocervical canal, but commonly covers part of the ectocervix.
- **Metaplasia** refers to the process by which columnar epithelium is replaced by squamous epithelium. It is stressed that this is a physiological process which occurs to a greater or lesser degree in all women. That part of the cervix which has been the site of metaplasia is recognizable colposcopically and is called the transformation zone.
- **Squamocolumnar junction** is the line of demarcation between columnar and squamous epithelium.
- **Leukoplakia** is a condition in which normal squamous epithelium is covered by a superficial cornified layer without visible nuclei. It is sometimes called **hyperkeratosis**.
- **Carcinoma-*in-situ*** is a lesion that exhibits atypical cells throughout the whole thickness of the squamous epithelium. Individually these cells are indistinguishable from those of invasive carcinoma but they do not breach the basement membrane, i.e. there is no invasion.
- **Dysplasia** represents a range of histological abnormalities between normal squamous epithelium and carcinoma-*in-situ*. The superficial cells are matured and fully differentiated but the underlying cells show atypical changes. Dysplasia is usually graded into mild, moderate and severe.
- **Cervical intraepithelial neoplasia (CIN)** is a new classification which many investigators find easier to use than dysplasia and carcinoma-*in-situ*. One of

its main advantages is that it removes the word carcinoma-*in-situ* from the terminology. There are three grades of CIN:

- – CIN1: equivalent to mild to moderate dysplasia;
- – CIN2: an intermediate grade;
- – CIN3: equivalent to severe dysplasia or carcinoma-*in-situ*.

- **Microinvasive carcinoma** is used if there is a minor degree of invasion. There is no generally accepted definition for this lesion, but most histopathologists would use the term if invasion was less than 4–5 mm below the basement membrane.
- **Invasive carcinoma** is present when there is unquestionable invasion by malignant cells.

COLPOSCOPIC TERMS

- **Acetowhite epithelium:** When 3% or 5% acetic acid is applied to the cervix, abnormal epithelium becomes white, with a sharp line of demarcation between the abnormal epithelium and the normal epithelium, which remains pink. In other words, acetowhite epithelium refers to that epithelium which is white **after** the application of acetic acid, in contradistinction to **leukoplakia**, which is white **before** the application of acetic acid.
- **Leukoplakia** or **hyperkeratosis** refers to epithelium that is white before the application of acetic acid. This can be seen with the naked eye.
- **Erosion** is mentioned here because, although it does not form part of the colposcopic terminology, it is commonly used in gynaecology. Colposcopic assessment of the cervix will show that a true erosion is an extremely rare occurrence, and when the gynaecologist describes the cervix as being the site of an erosion s/he usually means that it is red because of the presence of an ectopy (see below) or inflammation.
- **Ectopy** is used to denote the presence of columnar epithelium on the ecto-cervix. Such a cervix will appear red, particularly in pregnant women or those using the combined oral contraceptive, and a firmly taken cervical smear will often produce bleeding. An ectopy is not an abnormal finding and does not require treatment unless it is causing symptoms such as postcoital bleeding or excessive vaginal discharge.
- **Squamocolumnar junction (SCJ)** is the easily recognized junction between squamous epithelium (whether normal or abnormal) and columnar epithelium.
- **Typical transformation zone (TTZ):** This is the most important part of the cervix as far as the colposcopist is concerned. It refers to that part of the cervix which has been transformed by a process of metaplasia from columnar

epithelium to squamous epithelium. The transformation zone can be quite easily recognized by the presence of small gland openings, small Nabothian follicles and a typical subepithelial capillary pattern. It is important that the colposcopist should always inspect the transformation zone early and become familiar with its recognition. If the transformation zone is normal it is called 'typical transformation zone', whereas if there is any suggestion of abnormality it is called 'atypical transformation zone'.

- **Atypical transformation zone (ATZ)** refers to a transformation zone that shows epithelium with the characteristics of abnormality. The colposcopist would suspect the presence of abnormal epithelium if s/he sees the following:
    1. leukoplakia (hyperkeratosis);
    2. acetowhite epithelium;
    3. an abnormal subepithelial capillary pattern – punctation, mosaic or atypical vessels.

TECHNIQUE OF COLPOSCOPY

Several types of colposcopy are available, but all have the same basic property: to view the cervix at magnifications varying from ×6 to ×40. For colposcopy to be performed, the patient is placed in a modified lithotomy position. The cervix is exposed with a bivalve speculum, following which the epithelium is inspected. There are two basic schools of colposcopy: (i) that using classical or extended colposcopy; and (ii) that using the saline technique. Most people belong to the former school.

CLASSICAL OR EXTENDED COLPOSCOPY

This is the method advocated by the German school, and it is practised at most colposcopy centres. The cervix and upper vagina are first examined at magnifications of ×6, ×10 and ×16, following which excess mucus is removed from the cervix with a dry cotton-wool swab and the cervix is again inspected. If it is thought necessary to take a cervical smear it should be done at this stage, care being taken not to be too vigorous in the scraping, otherwise bleeding may occur and cause difficulties in interpreting the colposcopic findings. Routine smear-taking at the first visit is not always necessary because the colposcopist usually already knows that the cytology is abnormal – hence the referral to the colposcopy clinic.

ACETIC ACID TEST

Acetic acid (3% or 5%) is gently applied by means of a cotton-wool swab. The acetic acid is held in place for about 5 s, following which it is relatively easy to remove most of any remaining mucus. Abnormal epithelium (if present) now appears white (acetowhite epithelium) and almost invariably is very easy to distinguish from normal epithelium because of a sharp line of demarcation between the two. The normal squamous epithelium appears pink because the light from the colposcope picks up the redness of the subepithelial capillary pattern. Abnormal epithelium is white because the acetic acid coagulates protein in the nuclei and the cytoplasm; abnormal epithelium has a high nuclear density and therefore a high concentration of protein. This prevents light from passing through, the end result being that the subepithelial vessel pattern is less easy to see and the epithelium appears white. The higher the concentration of protein, the more intense will be the white appearance. The effect of the acetic acid wears off after about 30–40 s, but reappears after a further application. Following the application of the acetic acid, Schiller's iodine may be applied.

SCHILLER'S IODINE TEST

Normal squamous epithelium is characterized by an abundance of glycogen, whereas abnormal epithelium has relatively little. Application of Lugol's iodine solution to normal squamous epithelium will therefore produce a dark brown (almost black) stain, while columnar epithelium and abnormal epithelium, which contain little or no glycogen, remain unstained. Most experienced colposcopists do not use the Schiller's iodine test, although for the trainee colposcopist it is essential as occasionally milder forms of abnormality will be seen that would otherwise have remained undetected.

SALINE TECHNIQUE

Because the use of acetic acid or Lugol's iodine makes it difficult to study the angioarchitecture of the cervix, the saline technique was devised by Koller and developed by Kolstad, both working from the Norwegian Radium Hospital in Oslo. After the cervix has been exposed, mucus is gently removed with a cotton-wool swab and the cervix is moistened with physiological saline, which allows the subepithelial angioarchitecture to be studied in great detail. To see the capillaries clearly the use of a green filter and high magnification is advised, thus making the red capillaries appear darker and therefore stand out more clearly. The technique depends entirely on visualization of various vessel patterns and, although it is a much more difficult technique to master, it allows the colpo-scopist to predict the underlying histological pattern with great accuracy.

NORMAL AND ABNORMAL COLPOSCOPIC APPEARANCES

There are certain predictable features which the colposcopist must assess follow-ing the application of acetic acid and these can be summarized as follows:

1. vascular pattern;
2. intercapillary distance;
3. colour tone relative to the junction of normal and abnormal tissue;
4. surface pattern;
5. sharp line of demarcation between different types of epithelium.

Of these criteria, probably the most important are the vascular pattern and the intercapillary distance, and it is important that the colposcopist is thoroughly familiar with the different types of capillary that can be observed in the surface epithelium of normal and abnormal cervical epithelium.

VASCULAR PATTERN

Seen under the colposcope, the vascular pattern of normal squamous epithelium appears as fine dots or as a network of fine capillaries. Abnormal epithelium, on the other hand, has capillaries which are described as either punctation vessels, mosaic vessels or atypical vessels.

- **Punctation** is an easily recognized vascular pattern characterized by dilated, elongated and often twisted vessels arranged in a prominent punctate pattern.
- **Mosaic vessels** are arranged parallel to the surface in a characteristic mosaic or 'crazy-paving' pattern.
- **Atypical vessels** are capillaries that are very easily seen by the colposcopist. Typically they are irregular in size, shape, course and arrangement.

INTERCAPILLARY DISTANCE

The intercapillary distance is the distance between vessels or the space encom-passed by the mosaic vessels. The maximum intercapillary distance of normal capillaries varies, but is approximately 50–250 μm, with an average of 100 μm.

Colposcopic assessment of the intercapillary distance in abnormal epithelium is most easily done by comparing the abnormal capillaries with the capillaries of the adjacent normal squamous epithelium. The intercapillary distance in CIN and early invasive carcinoma of the cervix increases with the advancing grade of the lesion, i.e. in CIN1 lesions the average intercapillary distance may be 200 μm, whereas in CIN3 it is often 450–550 μm.

COLOUR TONE

When using the saline technique, abnormal epithelium appears much darker than normal epithelium, whereas following the application of acetic acid abnormal epithelium appears very white (acetowhite epithelium). In both cases, particularly following the application of acetic acid, an easily recognizable sharp line of demarcation between normal and abnormal epithelium can be observed.

SURFACE PATTERN

The surface of the lesion can be described as being smooth and even, granular, papillomatous or nodular. Normal squamous epithelium, for example, has a smooth surface, while columnar epithelium is easily recognized by its typical grape-like or villus appearance. At the other extreme invasive cancer is characterized by an uneven, nodular and often exophytic growth pattern.

LINES OF DEMARCATION

The line of demarcation between normal squamous epithelium and abnormal epithelium is usually sharp as a result of the change in colour that is present in abnormal epithelium.

APPENDIX C: BASIC COLPOSCOPY: MULTIPLE CHOICE QUESTIONS AND CLINICAL CASE SCENARIOS

ANSWERS TO MCQs

CHAPTER 1

1. The ectocervical native epithelium is:
    a. Of columnar mucinous type.   False
    b. Resistant to hormone effects.   False
    c. Of multilayered squamous type.   True
    d. Commonly ulcerated.   False
    e. Very fragile in comparison to the endocervical epithelium. False

2. The 'physiological' squamocolumnar junction:
    a. Is where the squamous and endocervical epithelium met in
       childhood.   False
    b. Is a fixed point.   False
    c. Moves under the influence of hormones.   True
    d. Is usually well within the endocervical canal in the pre-
       menopausal woman.   False
    e. Does not exist.   False

3. The transformation zone:
    a. Is where native endocervical epithelium has been converted to
       squamous epithelium.   True
    b. Is no longer present in post-menopausal women.   False
    c. Never has underlying crypts.   False
    d. Never contains crypt openings.   False

4. **Squamous metaplasia is not:**
   a. A physiological process. False
   b. Brought about by the effect of vaginal acidity. False
   c. Stimulated by trauma. False
   d. Caused by human papillomaviruses. True
   e. Preceded by reserve cell hyperplasia. False

5. **The congenital transformation zone is:**
   a. Formed post-menopausally. False
   b. Related to uterine fundal abnormalities. False
   c. Formed in pre-natal or early post-natal life. True
   d. Often associated with excess epithelial glycogen production. False
   e. Invisible colposcopically. False

CHAPTER 2

6. **With regard to cervical smear-taking and reporting:**
   a. The person taking the smear usually decides if the sample is adequate. False
   b. A smear report of moderate dyskaryosis should be managed as for mild dyskaryosis. False
   c. The transformation zone is difficult to sample in post-menopausal patients. True
   d. Colposcopy is not indicated following a smear report of abnormal endocervical cells. False
   e. Cervical cytology can reliably detect invasive squamous cell cancer. False

CHAPTER 3

7. **The following histological features distinguish CIN3 from CIN1:**
   a. CIN3 shows greater nuclear pleomorphism than CIN1. True
   b. CIN3 shows greater variation in nuclear size than CIN1. True
   c. CIN3 shows better differentiation than CIN1. False
   d. Nuclei at the surface are normal in CIN1. False
   e. Nucleoli are more prominent in CIN1 than in CIN3. False

8. **Which of the following statements about CGIN are true?**
   a. CGIN naturally falls into three categories. False
   b. The term high-grade CGIN includes adenocarcinoma-*in-situ*. True

   c. There is a clear progression from low-grade CGIN to
      adenocarcinoma.   False
   d. Cervical crypts may be involved by all grades of GGIN.   True
   e. CGIN is best excised using LLETZ.   False

9. **The following are histological features of early invasive carcinoma:**
   a. Focal lymphocytic infiltrate in the stroma.   True
   b. Anaplasia of the invasive cells.   False
   c. Eosinophilia of the invasive cells.   True
   d. Ulceration of the surface epithelium.   False
   e. Focal condensation of stromal collagen.   False

CHAPTER 4

10. **With regard to the history of colposcopy:**
   a. Colposcopy was introduced by Hans Hinselmann.   True
   b. Colposcopy is complementary to cervical cytology.   True
   c. Commonly used magnifications are up to 200-fold.   False
   d. The focal length varies between 200 and 300 mm.   True
   e. The blue filter has been an important development in the
      field of colposcopy.   False

11. **With regard to equipment in the colposcopy clinic:**
   a. The smallest speculum available should be used.   False
   b. Iris hooks can be useful for manipulation.   True
   c. Lugol's iodine is a useful stain to detect pre-invasive disease.   True
   d. An endocervical speculum is useful for examining the lower
      endocervical canal.   True
   e. Biopsies should be taken randomly from the cervical
      transformation zone.   False

12. **During a colposcopic examination:**
   a. The cervix should be partially exposed.   False
   b. Assessment of the angioarchitecture is important.   True
   c. Normal squamous epithelium fails to stain with acetic acid.   True
   d. Areas of metaplasia are abnormal, and should be excised.   False
   e. Acetowhite lesions extending onto the vagina may be
      encountered in some instances.   True

CHAPTER 5

13. **Regarding metaplasia:**
    a. Immature metaplasia stains white following acetic acid.   True
    b. A high vaginal pH causes squamous epithelium to change to
       columnar.   False
    c. Columnar epithelium cannot be present within the
       transformation zone.   False
    d. Fusion of villi in columnar epithelium is an early metaplastic
       event.   False
    e. The metaplastic process is patchy, uneven and irregular in
       timing.   True

14. **Regarding colposcopy:**
    a. Colposcopy cannot differentiate between original squamous
       and metaplastic epithelium.   False
    b. Gland openings confirm that the epithelium is original
       squamous epithelium.   False
    c. The distal limit of the transformation zone is usually easy to
       define.   True
    d. Double capillaries usually indicate an inflammatory process.   True
    e. Lugol's iodine is useful to study the vascular patterns on the
       cervix.   False

CHAPTER 6

15. **The following are indications for colposcopy in the UK:**
    a. A single mildly dyskaryotic smear.   False
    b. A single moderately dyskaryotic smear.   True
    c. A single severely dyskaryotic smear.   True
    d. A cervical polyp.   False
    e. A routine follow-up visit 18 months after treatment for CIN3. False

16. **Which of the following statements are true?**
    a. There is a high correlation between negative cytology and
       negative histology.   True
    b. There is a high correlation between low-grade cytology and
       low-grade histology.   False
    c. There is a high correlation between high-grade cytology and
       high-grade histology.   True
    d. HPV 16 is a high-risk oncogenic virus.   True
    e. HPV 6 is a high-risk oncogenic virus.   False

17. **Which of the following statements about colposcopy are true?**
    a. It was first developed in Germany. — True
    b. It is used as a screening tool in some genitourinary medicine clinics in the UK. — True
    c. It is usually performed at a magnification of ×40. — False
    d. It is only used to examine female anatomy. — False
    e. It is essential in the diagnosis of VIN. — False

CHAPTER 7

18. **Acetowhite change may be seen in the following conditions:**
    a. CIN. — True
    b. Wart virus infection. — True
    c. Metaplasia. — True
    d. Invasive squamous carcinoma. — True
    e. Congenital transformation zone. — True

19. **If atypical blood vessels are seen on colposcopy:**
    a. A punch biopsy is required to rule out invasion. — False
    b. The lesion may be treated with cold coagulation. — False
    c. This gives rise to suspicion of an invasive lesion. — True
    d. They may be ignored if the smear shows mild dyskaryosis. — False
    e. They are commonly seen on the surface of Nabothian follicles. — False

20. **CIN:**
    a. Can always be diagnosed on colposcopy. — False
    b. Can be diagnosed with the naked eye. — False
    c. Is never found in association with condyloma accuminata of the cervix. — False
    d. Can be diagnosed with a colposcope without use of acetic acid. — True
    e. Is excluded if the smear is normal. — False

CHAPTER 8

21. **Regarding HGCGIN:**
    a. Patients usually present with abnormal bleeding. — False
    b. It has well-defined colposcopic features. — False
    c. Cone biopsy is only useful as a diagnostic procedure. — False
    d. Frequently presents with coexistent squamous lesions. — True
    e. Pregnancy changes may mask the usual colposcopic features. — False

22. **The following statements are true:**
    a. When glandular lesions are suspected, excisional biopsy must be performed.   False
    b. When frank invasion is apparent, diagnostic cone biopsy is mandatory.   False
    c. Coarse punctation is a typical feature of HGCGIN.   False
    d. Early invasive lesions are likely to have wide intercapillary distances.   True
    e. Acetic acid application can mask abnormal vascular patterns.   False

23. **Regarding early invasive lesions:**
    a. Cervical cytology is highly predictive.   False
    b. Knife cone is best avoided.   False
    c. Patients with Stage Ia$_2$ disease should be referred to a cancer centre for further management.   True
    d. Local treatment, using ablation, is acceptable.   False

CHAPTER 9

24. **Recording information in colposcopy clinics:**
    a. The number of previous sexual partners is an essential part of the colposcopy minimum dataset.   False
    b. The minimum dataset records the findings of bimanual examination at the first attendance.   False
    c. Photography is useful in assessing the extent of involvement of the vaginal angles in VaIN.   False
    d. The patient's hospital number is the preferred unique identifier. False
    e. The use of digital image capture has no proven benefits in managing patients in the colposcopy clinic.   True

25. **In colpophotography:**
    a. A beam-splitting device attached to the colposcopes reduces the light intensity.   True
    b. Black and white film (enhanced by the addition of a red filter) is better for recording vascular architecture.   False
    c. Videophotography gives better depth of focus than still photography.   False
    d. Cervicographs are assessed by an expert, who examines the projected slide of the cervix at a fixed distance.   True
    e. A film speed of 400 ASA is ideal for photographing the cervix. False

CHAPTER 10

26. **Epidemiology:**
    a. The incidence of cervical cancer continues to decline.   True
    b. Cervical cancer is the commonest female cancer worldwide.   False
    c. Approximately 11% of all cervical smears taken are abnormal to some degree.   False
    d. Almost 10% of smears taken in the UK are reported as unsatisfactory.   True
    e. Almost 6 million smears are performed annually in the UK.   False

27. **Patient selection:**
    a. All cases of CIN must undergo immediate treatment.   False
    b. A colposcopic-directed punch biopsy should always be taken in women with abnormal cervical cytology.   False
    c. A colposcopic-directed punch biopsy can be helpful in assessing the degree of abnormality.   True
    d. High-grade CIN in pregnancy should be immediately treated.   False
    e. Young women with low-grade CIN may be managed conservatively.   True

28. **Non-treatment of cytological abnormalities:**
    a. If there is no lesion present at colposcopy, the woman should be discharged to routine screening.   False
    b. Women with CIN3 have a lower progressive potential than those with CIN1.   False
    c. HPV testing may predict those women with high-grade CIN.   True
    d. HPV testing may allow selection of those women requiring colposcopy among those with equivocal cytological abnormalities.   True
    e. CIN has a centripetal distribution (i.e. higher-grade CIN is centrally placed in a lesion).   True

CHAPTER 11

29. **In the treatment of CIN:**
    a. Excision and ablation are both appropriate in recurrent cases.   False
    b. All methods other than hysterectomy require prior colposcopy.   False
    c. Before ablation, a directed biopsy should be performed.   True
    d. Loop excision can be used to 'see-and-treat' without recourse to biopsy.   True
    e. Local anaesthetic is injected into the TZ prior to excision.   False

30. **The following situations require a biopsy:**
    a. Mild dyskaryosis in a 22-year-old with normal satisfactory colposcopy. False
    b. Two borderline smears in a 28-year-old previously treated for CIN2. True
    c. Suspected CIN1 in pregnancy. False
    d. Cervical smear in a 40-year-old reported as glandular atypia. True
    e. Mild dyskaryosis in a 60-year-old with leukoplakia on the cervix. True

31. **Treatment of CIN should not be performed:**
    a. In pregnancy. True
    b. If there is an acute vaginal infection. True
    c. In the luteal phase. False
    d. During menstruation. False
    e. In women who are HIV-positive. False

CHAPTER 12

32. **After local ablative or excisional treatment of CIN:**
    a. The risk of frank invasive cancer is greater than in 1000. True
    b. Most residual disease will be recognized within 12 months. True
    c. Colposcopy and cytology should be performed within 3 months. False
    d. Recurrent disease is more likely than residual disease. False
    e. A success rate of between 90% and 95% can be expected. True

33. **Follow-up for treated CIN:**
    a. Includes colposcopy at 12 months in all women. False
    b. Is more likely to be abnormal in women who have had high-grade lesions treated. True
    c. Is based on colposcopy rather than cytology. False
    d. May be normal despite the presence of residual disease. True
    e. Requires an annual smear for 3 years. False

34. **After a hysterectomy:**
    a. Women who have never had an abnormal smear require no further cytological surveillance. True
    b. Colposcopy and cytology should be performed at 6 weeks. False
    c. Colposcopy and cytology should be a part of follow-up if CIN is present. True
    d. There is a risk of vaginal intraepithelial neoplasia (VaIN) in all patients. False

e. Lugol's iodine is more reliable in detecting residual CIN than acetic acid. False

35. **In untreated patients with abnormal smears:**
    a. Colposcopy may be normal despite a moderately dyskaryotic smear. True
    b. The preferred treatment for persistent dyskaryosis is ablation. False
    c. Two consecutively negative smears are required prior to discharge back to routine recall. True
    d. Random punch biopsies should be performed if colposcopy is normal. False
    e. A normal punch biopsy means that the patient can be discharged to recall. False

CHAPTER 13

36. **Early, invasive squamous cell carcinoma of the cervix may be defined as:**
    a. A lesion with a volume of <300 mm^3. True
    b. A lesion invading up to 5 mm into the basement membrane. True
    c. A lesion on the cervix which is invisible to the naked eye. False
    d. A lesion 2 mm deep and 8 mm wide. False

37. **Fertility-sparing surgery may be considered in:**
    a. Stage Ia cervical cancer. True
    b. Stage Ib cervical cancer. True
    c. Adenocarcinoma-*in-situ*. True
    d. A patient with a recurrent severely dyskaryotic smear after LLETZ for CIN3. True

38. **Adenocarcinoma of the cervix:**
    a. Is decreasing in incidence. False
    b. Has a defined microinvasive precursor lesion. False
    c. Has a defined '*in-situ*' precursor lesion. True
    d. Is found in nearly all cases in conjunction with an invasive squamous lesion. False

39. **FIGO criteria used to define microinvasive squamous cell carcinoma include:**
    a. Depth of invasion. True
    b. Tumour volume. False
    c. Tumour area. True
    d. The colposcopic appearance of the lesion. False

40. **Radical trachelectomy:**
    a. Is associated with a poorer long-term outcome than radical
       hysterectomy.   False
    b. Should only be considered in women with no children.   False
    c. Includes bilateral uterine artery ligation.   False
    d. Does not allow such a large vaginal cuff to be removed.   False

CHAPTER 14

41. **Regarding HPV and CIN, are the following statements true or false?**
    a. The prevalence of HPV infection in the normal female
       population is approximately 15%.   True
    b. Hybrid capture is useful in mass screening.   True
    c. Quantitative HPV testing is as sensitive as cytology in detecting
       high-grade cervical disease.   False
    d. Viral load is important in predicting future cervical disease.   True
    e. Vaccines currently have a role to play in CIN prevention.   False

CHAPTER 15

42. **During pregnancy:**
    a. CIN is less likely to progress to cancer.   False
    b. Atypical features in the TZ are more obvious.   False
    c. Treatment of CIN should be avoided.   True
    d. Directed punch biopsy is the preferred method of excluding
       invasion.   False
    e. Acetic acid should not be used.   False

43. **With regard to the menopause:**
    a. Hormone replacement therapy (HRT) may help to cause
       metaplasia.   False
    b. Local oestrogen may help to improve the quality of cytology.   True
    c. Schiller's test is of more value than in the pre-menopausal state. False
    d. Cervical screening can now be discontinued.   False
    e. Taking a smear can result in inadequate colposcopy.   True

44. **A pathology report of incomplete excision:**
    a. Means that there is a greater risk of persistent disease.   True
    b. Means that further treatment is required.   False
    c. Can be managed by either laser or another suitable ablative
       technique.   False

    d. Requires a directed punch biopsy if microinvasion has been
       reported.   False
    e. Can be followed up by cytology in the community.   False

CHAPTER 16

45. **In viral infections of the cervix:**
    a. A wart virus infection reported on a cervical smear is an
       indication for colposcopy.   False
    b. Cervical cytology is highly specific in diagnosing HSV.   False
    c. Women with a past history of genital HSV should have annual
       cervical cytology.   False
    d. Warts on the cervix stain white with acetic acid.   True
    e. HPV 16 and 18 infection demonstrates an acetowhite
       response; HPV 6 and 11 do not.   False

46. **In sexually transmitted diseases:**
    a. The 'strawberry cervix' is suggestive of *Trichomonas*
       vaginalis infection.   True
    b. *Gardnerella vaginalis* causes irregular branching of
       subepithelial capillaries, giving a classical colposcopic
       appearance.   False
    c. The pathognomonic cytological indication of HSV is the 'foam
       cell'.   True
    d. Exophytic cervical warts are an indication for annual cervical
       cytology.   False
    e. Some 5% of deaths from squamous carcinoma of the cervix
       in the UK occur in HIV-positive women.   False

47. **With regard to HIV-positive women:**
    a. The prevalence of high-grade dysplasia in HIV-positive women
       is estimated to be between 20% and 50%.   True
    b. HIV-positive women are more often infected with HPV than
       HIV-negative women.   True
    c. The prevalence of cervical dysplasia increases as immuno-
       suppression advances.   True
    d. Dysplasia amongst HIV-positive women is four times more
       likely to progress than in HIV-negative women.   True
    e. The prevalence of dysplasia in HIV-positive women increases
       with higher viral load measurement, even if the CD4 cell count
       remains stable.   True

CHAPTER 17

48. **When counselling women, are the following true or false?**

    a. Women waiting for a colposcopy examination are more anxious than those awaiting major surgery.   True

    b. A full sexual history should always be taken as part of a woman's colposcopy assessment.   False

    c. Detailed information booklets are most effective in reducing anxiety.   False

    d. A 'see-and-treat' policy is less anxiety-provoking than a 'select-and-treat' policy for women.   False

    e. The large majority of women with CIN1 left untreated would not develop cervical cancer.   True

    f. Simple written information specific to each colposcopy unit is as effective as video information.   False

    g. Up to 70% of women will test positive for genital HPV infection at some stage in their reproductive life.   True

ANSWERS TO CLINICAL CASE SCENARIO QUESTIONS

CLINICAL CASE SCENARIO 1

A 22-year-old para 0+0 is referred for colposcopy with a smear showing mild dyskaryosis on two occasions. On colposcopic examination, an initial assessment reveals no abnormality.

Acetic acid (5%) is applied to reveal the following:

- The whole TZ is seen.
- The anterior lip of the cervix reveals faint acetowhite epithelium grade I, with a faint edge to the ectocervical margin of the TZ.
- There is a mosaic pattern of the vessels.
- The posterior lip reveals the acetowhite change to be more dense (grade II), with clear evidence of mosaic pattern of blood vessels.
- There are no abnormal vessels.

Questions

1. What do the colposcopic findings suggest?
2. Is this compatible with the smear report?
3. What is the minimum number of biopsies that should be taken?

4. Does the appearance suggest an invasive lesion?
5. What form of treatments may be appropriate when biopsy results are available?

Answers

1. The initial referral smear of mild dyskaryosis on two occasions warrants referral for colposcopic review. Some units will accept referral with one smear showing mild dyskaryosis.
2. The colposcopic features suggest possible differing histology on the anterior and posterior lips of the cervix. The features on the anterior lip are compatible with viral change alone, but do not rule out CIN. The more intense acetowhite appearance of the posterior lip are more in keeping with CIN, but histology is required to confirm this.
3. A minimum of two punch biopsies should be taken; the anterior and posterior lips should be biopsied.
4. The statement that no abnormal vessels are present along with the features confirms no evidence of invasive disease.
5. Once histology is known and confirms CIN of a major grade, the lesion may be treated by excision or ablation of the transformation zone, as the whole area of abnormality can be seen. The former method is now much more common in UK practice as further tissue may be assessed histologically. If biopsy shows minor grade CIN with viral change, there still remains debate regarding the requirements for treatment. Future HPV testing for oncogenic types may resolve this. However, no matter whether treatment or observation is proposed, follow-up is essential.

CLINICAL CASE SCENARIO 2

A 46-year-old patient presented with a 'positive' glandular smear, suggestive of endocervical carcinoma. She was asymptomatic and had regular, normal periods. Her previous cervical smears had been normal. She was nulliparous and a non-smoker. She needed no contraception but had been on the oral contraceptive 'pill' in the past. Colposcopy was unremarkable; the examination was satisfactory, the squamocolumnar junction was seen, and no abnormality was noted. Bimanual examination was normal. After discussion, an endometrial sample and an extended loop diathermy cone was performed. Histology was requested urgently and the specimen was found to contain HGCGIN. There was no evidence of invasive cancer, but it was not possible to be sure that the HGCGIN had been completely excised. The endometrial sample was normal. The options were discussed, which ranged from cytological follow-up to hysterectomy. Further excision was advised and the patient opted for knife conization. This specimen contained no residual disease and arrangements were made for follow-up in the colpscopy clinic in 6 months' time.

Questions

1. How urgently should patients with smears such as this be seen? What investigations are appropriate? How do women with CGIN normally present?
2. What factors have been implicated in the aetiology of CGIN?
3. What is the most appropriate biopsy for suspected CGIN, and why?
4. Is bimanual examination always necessary in women referred with such smears? If so why does this differ from the norm?
5. What is the rationale for the types of acceptable management?

Answers

1. Patients with smears suggestive of high-grade glandular abnormality should be managed as if dealing with cancer, i.e. seen within 14 days. One needs to consider the possibility of other glandular cancers within the genital tract, including the endometrium and ovaries. Most patients with CGIN present with abnormal smears, many of which will show squamous abnormalities.
2. The aetiology and natural history of CGIN is not understood. There is a statistical association between the oral contraceptive pill and cervical adeno-carcinoma. As for squamous lesions, there is an association between cervical glandular neoplasia and HPV infection.
3. In the presence of a high-grade glandular lesion an excisional diagnositic biopsy of the cervix is necessary. The biopsy size and shape will be influenced by the colposcopic findings, but must include an adequate sampling of the endocervical canal. The biopsy should aim to be therapeutic, with a length of at least 25 mm. Diathermy conization is easy, practical and avoids the use of general anaethesia, though assessment of excision margins can be difficult.
4. As a rule, bimanual vaginal examinations are not part of routine colposcopy. However, when dealing with suspected malignancy, such an examination should be considered.
5. Management depends on a variety of considerations. Conization alone has been shown to be an acceptable form of treatment, provided that the resection margins are uninvolved. On the other hand, hysterectomy is also an option as there are theoretical concerns about 'skip' lesions and the adequacy of cytological follow-up, which must include endocervical smears.

CLINICAL CASE SCENARIO 3

A 22-year-old nulliparous woman attended for her first ever cervical smear. She enjoyed good general health and had no gynaecological symptoms. The cervical smear was reported as showing mildly dyskaryotic changes.

Questions

1. Should this woman be referred for immediate colposcopic assessment?
2. Follow-up showed mild dyskaryosis and colposcopy was consistent with HGCIN. Should the patient undergo immediate LLETZ?
3. Following treatment, is the woman at increased risk of invasive cervical cancer?

Answers

1. If the patient is deemed likely to default from cytological surveillance, then arrangements should be made for immediate colposcopic assessment and possible treatment. However, if the woman is amenable to surveillance, then the cervical smear should be repeated after an interval of six months. Another option would be to test for the oncogenic HPV types to help predict the presence of high-grade CIN.

   [The cervical smear was repeated after an interval of 6 months, and similar cytological changes were again detected. On referral for colposcopic assessment, a clinical impression of high-grade intraepithelial neoplasia was suggested.]

2. Approximately one-third of patients with mildly dyskaryotic cervical smears will have high-grade intraepithelial neoplasia. However, colposcopy may overcall the lesion and in this circumstance taking account of her age and nulliparity, it might be helpful to confirm the diagnosis prior to proceeding to definitive treatment.

   [Two punch biopsies from the cervical transformation zone were taken, and these confirmed the presence of CIN3. In view of this, arrangements were made for her to undergo LLETZ to remove the abnormality. Follow-up cervical cytology reverted to normal at the 6-month post-treatment assessment.]

3. Any woman who has been treated for CIN remains at a higher risk than the general population for invasive cervical disease. In those women where the smear reverts back to normal, this risk is of the order of two to three times the background risk. In those with abnormal cervical cytology following treatment, then the risk of invasive disease is significant (25 to 30 times) compared with the general population.

CLINICAL CASE SCENARIO 4

A 39-year-old woman, para 2+1, attended for colposcopy after a moderately dyskaryotic smear. Colposcopy revealed an acetowhite area on the posterior cervical lip which was considered to be CIN2, and LLETZ was carried out. Histology revealed squamous carcinoma-*in-situ* and also an adenocarcinoma-*in-situ*. The ectocervical margin was normal, but there were adenocarcinoma cells at the endocervical margin.

Questions

1. How should this patient's management proceed?
2. The upper margin of the specimen was positive and a further cervical specimen was required; this confirmed AIS, with negative margins. Six months later the cervix was colposcopically normal and a smear was taken that showed normal squamous cells only, with no metaplastic or endocervical cells. How should her management proceed?
3. In this case, the endocervical canal has not been sampled and the patient should be recalled. How can this be best achieved?
4. How can the endocervical canal be evaluated, given that unfortunately the cytology is still unsatisfactory?

Answers

1. Since the upper margin of the specimen is positive, there is the possibility of an invasive lesion. Therefore, a further cervical specimen is required. This may be obtained by a formal knife cone biopsy.
2. The second specimen confirmed AIS, with negative margins. No further action was taken, and the woman was reviewed in the colposcopy clinic 6 months later. At that visit, the cervix was colposcopically normal and a smear was taken. This showed normal squamous cells only, with no metaplastic or endocervical cells.
3. In order to recall the patient it would be advisable to speak to her directly or inform her in a letter as to why you are recalling her – she will, rightly, be very concerned as to why she is being asked to visit the colposcopy clinic early. However she is contacted, it should be explained that the endocervical canal needs to be sampled. The accuracy of a canal smear taken with a cytobrush seems as good as that taken at endocervical curettage.
4. The os could be dilated under general anaesthesia, which might improve the cervical stenosis. (At the same time, the endocervix could be sampled with a curette.) Microhysteroscopy might be attempted (as a 'surgery' procedure, under local anaesthetic), or the canal can be evaluated with

vaginal ultrasonography. If the endocervix remains impossible to sample, and especially if a further abnormal smear is obtained or if the patient develops associated gynaecological symptoms which could well be treated with hysterectomy, then this should be considered. Of course, the patient may request this if she has sufficient anxiety regarding prognosis/inadequate cytology.

CLINICAL CASE SCENARIO 5

Emily is a 38-year-old African woman who is applying for asylum in this country. She is known to be HIV-positive, and has a CD4 cell count under 100, with a viral load of more than 400 000 copies per ml.

Adherence to her antiretroviral treatment is episodic, and in the past she has been treated for *Pneumocystis carinii* pneumonia and syphilis. Cervical cytology has been performed in the GUM department, where severe dyskaryosis was found and colposcopy performed. The colposcopic appearance was suggestive of high-grade CIN, and biopsies showed CIN3 with HPV; the squamocolumnar junction was not visible. Cone biopsy was advised.

Questions

1. Do smears from women attending GUM departments have a higher likelihood of any significant abnormality being found?
2. Do women with HIV have a higher incidence of cervical dysplasia?
3. Are women who are immunosuppressed at increased risk for acquiring HPV infection?
4. Is cone biopsy contraindicated in women such as this with significant immunosuppression and HIV seropositivity?

Answers

1. Analysis of cervical smear results compared with the clinic of origin show that whilst there is a small increase in the likelihood of borderline and mildly dyskaryotic smears occurring in GUM clinics, there is **not** an increased likelihood for moderate or worse dyskaryosis. This may be partly explained by the increased percentage of GUM cytologies being from younger women.
2. Women with HIV are 10 times more likely to have abnormal cytology on routine screening, with up to 40% of HIV-positive women having cervical dysplasia.
3. Women who are immunosuppressed are at increased risk for acquiring HPV infection. HIV-positive women with CD4 cell counts below 200 are more

than 10 times as likely as HIV-negative women, to have HPV infection. Women with HIV are three times as likely to be infected with more than one subtype of HPV as is their HPV-infected, HIV-negative 'sister'.

4. HIV positivity *per se* is not a reason for not treating such women. Adherence to antiretroviral treatment could result in rapid and effective immunoreconstruction and improvement in general health. CIN may regress in conjunction with this, but this cannot be relied upon. Continued immunosuppression following treatment is a risk factor for CIN recurrence.

APPENDIX D:
FURTHER READING

CHAPTER 1

Fu, Y.S. and Reagan, J.W. 1989: Development, anatomy and histology of the lower female genital tract. In: *Pathology of the Uterine Cervix, Vagina and Vulva*. Philadelphia: Saunders, p. 21.

Singer, A. and Jordan, J.A. 1976: The anatomy of the cervix. In: Jordan, J.A. and Singer, A., eds. *The Cervix*. London: Saunders, p. 13.

Ferenczy, A. and Winkler, B. 1994: Anatomy and histology of the cervix. In: Kurman, R., ed. *Blaustein's Pathology of the Female Genital Tract*, 4th edn. New York: Springer-Verlag, p. 185.

CHAPTER 2

Koss, L.G. 1989: The Papanicolaou test for cervical cancer: a triumph and a tragedy. *Journal of the American Medical Association* **261**, 734–743.

Evans, D. M. D., Hudson, E. A., Brown, C. L. *et al.* 1986: Terminology on gynaecological cytopathology: report of the working party of the BSCC. *Journal of Clinical Pathology* **39**, 933–944.

Wied, G. L., Keebler, C. M., Koss, L. G. *et al.* 1992: *Compendium of Diagnostic Pathology*, Tutorials of Cytology, Chicago, IL.

CHAPTER 3

Anderson, M.C. 1995: Premalignant and malignant squamous lesions of the cervix. In: Fox, H. and Wells, M, eds. *Haines and Taylor Obstetrical and Gynaecological Pathology*, 4th edn, Churchill Livingstone, Edinburgh.

Anderson, M.C., Brown, C.L., Fox, H. *et al.* 1991: Current views on cervical intraepithelial neoplasia. *Journal of Clinical Pathology* **44**, 969–978.

Histopathology Reporting in Cervical Screening. Report of the Working Party of The Royal College of Pathologists and the NHS Cervical Screening Programme. Chairman: H. Fox. NHSCSP Publication No.10. April 1999.

Wright, T.C., Kurman, R.J. and Ferenczy, A. 1994: Precancerous lesions of the cervix. In: Kurman, R.J., ed. *Blaustein's Pathology of the Female Genital Tract*, 4th edn, Springer, New York.

CHAPTER 4

Jordan, J.A. 1985: Colposcopy in the diagnosis of cervical cancer and precancer. *Clinical Obstetrics and Gynecology* **12**, 67–76.

Soutter, W.P. 1991: Criteria for standards of management of women with an abnormal smear. *British Journal of Obstetrics and Gynaecology* **98**, 1069–1072.

Stafl, A. 1983: Understanding colposcopic patterns and their clinical significance. *Contemporary Obstetrics and Gynaecology* **21**, 85–104.

CHAPTER 6

Duncan, I.D. (ed.) 1992: *Guidelines For Clinical Practice and Programme Management*. NHS Cervical Screening Programme National Co-ordinating Network, Oxford.

Duncan, I.D. (ed.) 1997: *Guidelines For Clinical Practice and Programme Management*, 2nd edition. NHSCSP Publications, Sheffield.

Jarmulowicz, M.R., Jenkins, D., Barton, S.E., Goodall, A.L., Hollingworth, A., Singer, A. 1989: Cytological status and lesion size. A further dimension in cervical intraepithelial neoplasia. *British Journal of Obstetrics and Gynaecology* **96**, 1061–1066.

Jordan, J.A., Sharp, F., Singer, A. (eds) 1981: *Pre-Clinical Neoplasia of The Cervix. Proceedings of the 9th Study Group*. London: Royal College of Obstetricians and Gynaecologists.

Lyall, H., Duncan, I.D. 1995: Inaccuracy of cytologic diagnosis in high grade squamous intraepithelial lesions (CIN3). *Acta Cytologica* **39**, 50–54.

CHAPTER 8

Anderson, M.C. 1993: Invasive carcinoma of the cervix following local destructive treatment for cervical intraepithelial neoplasia. *British Journal of Obstetrics and Gynaecology* **100**, 657–663.

Benedet, J., Anderson, G. and Boyes, D. 1985: Colposcopic accuracy in the diagnosis of microinvasive and occult invasive carcinoma of the cervix. *Obstetrics and Gynecology* **65**, 557–562.

Luesley, D., Cullimore, J., Redman, C. *et al.* 1990: Loop diathermy excision of the cervical transformation zone in patients with abnormal cervical smears. *British Medical Journal* **300**, 1690–1693.

Shafi, M., Finn, C., Luesley, D. *et al.* 1991: Lesion size and histology of atypical transformation zone. *British Journal of Obstetrics and Gynaecology* **98**, 490–492.

Shafi, M., Dunn, J., Chenoy, R. *et al.* 1994: Digital imaging colposcopy, image analysis, and quantification of the colposcopic image. *British Journal of Obstetrics and Gynaecology* **97**, 811–816.

CHAPTER 9

Shafi, M., Dunn, J., Chenoy, R. *et al.* 1994: Digital imaging colposcopy, image analysis, and quantification of the colposcopic image. *British Journal of Obstetrics and Gynaecology* **97**, 811–816.

Soutter, W.P. 1991: Criteria for standards of measurement of women with an abnormal smear. *British Journal of Obstetrics and Gynaecology* **98**, 1069–1072.

Stafl, A. 1981: Cervicography: a new method for cervical cancer detection. *American Journal of Obstetrics and Gynecology* **139**, 815–825.

CHAPTER 10

Duncan, I.D. 1992: *Guidelines for Clinical Practice and Programme Management*, NHS Cervical Screening Programme National Co-ordinating Network, Oxford.

Richart, R.M. 1990: A modified terminology for cervical intraepithelial neoplasia. *Obstetrics and Gynecology* **75**, 131–133.

Royal College of Obstetricians and Gynaecologists 1987: *Report of the Intercollegiate Working Party on Cervical Screening*, RCOG, London.

CHAPTER 12

Duncan, I.D. 1992: *Guidelines for Clinical Practice and Programme Management*, NHS Cervical Screening Programme National Co-ordinating Network, Oxford.

Kitchener, H.C., Cruickshank, M.C. and Farmery, E. 1995: The 1993 BSCCP/NCN United Kingdom Colposcopy Survey: comparison with 1988 and the response to introduction of guidelines. *British Journal of Obstetrics and Gynaecology* **102**(7), 549–552.

Lopes, A., Mor Yosef, S., Pearson, S. *et al.* 1990: Is routine colposcopic assessment necessary following laser ablation of cervical intraepithelial neoplasia? *British Journal of Obstetrics and Gynaecology* **97**, 175–177.

Paraskevaidis, E., Jandial, L., Mann E. *et al.* 1991: Pattern of treatment failure following laser for cervical intraepithelial neoplasia: implications for follow-up. *Obstetrics and Gynecology* **78**, 883.

CHAPTER 13

Nahhas, W., Sharkey, F. and Whitney, C. 1983: The prognostic significance of vascular channel involvement in deep stroma penetration in early cervical carcinoma. *American Journal of Clinical Oncology*, **6**, 259.

Shingleton, H.M., Gore, H., Bradley, D.H. and Soong, S.-J. 1981: Adenocarcinoma of the cervix. I: Clinical evaluation and pathological features. *American Journal of Obstetrics and Gynecology*, **139**, 799.

Van Nagell, J., Jr, Greenwell, N., Powell, D. and Donaldson, E. 1983: Microinvasive carcinoma of the cervix. *American Journal of Obstetrics and Gynecology*, **145**, 981.

Shepherd, J.H., Crawford, R.A.F. and Oram, D.H. 1998: Radical trachelectomy: a way to preserve fertility in the treatment of early cervical cancer. *British Journal of Obstetrics and Gynaecology*, **105**, 912.

CHAPTER 16

Moss, T. and Hicks, D.A. 1994: *The Role of Genito-urinary Medicine Cytology and Colposcopy in Cervical Screening*. NHS Cervical Screening Programme: definitive document.

Paavonen, J., Stevens, C.E., Wølner-Hanssen, P. *et al.* 1988: Colposcopic manifestations of cervical and vaginal infections. *Obstetric and Gynaecological Survey* **43**(7), 373–381.

CHAPTER 17

Austoker, J., Davey, C. and Jansen, C. 1997: *Improving the quality of written information sent to women about cervical screening: Guidelines on the Presentation and content of letters and leaflets*. NHSCSP Publication No 5.

Doherty, I.E. and Richardson, P.H. 1995: Psychological aspects of the investigation and treatment of abnormalities of the cervix. In: Luesley, D.M., Jordan, J. and Richart, R.M., eds. *Intraepithelial Neoplasm of the Lower Genital Tract*, Chapter 19. Edinburgh: Churchill Livingstone.

Posner, T. 1998: The psychosocial impact of cervical intraepithelial neoplasia and its management. In: Luesley, D.M. and Barrasso, R., eds. *Cancer and Pre-cancer of the Cervix*, Chapter 12. London: Chapman & Hall.

Posner, T. and Vessey, M. 1988: *Prevention of Cervical Cancer: The Patient's View*. King Edward's Hospital Fund for London.

INDEX

Note: MCQ are in bold; clinical scenarios are in italics. Page numbers in brackets following clinical scenario page numbers indicate answers to questions. Abbreviations: CGIN, cervical glandular intraepithelial; CIN, cervical intraepithelial neoplasia; GUM, genitourinary medicine; TZ, transformation zone; VaIB, vaginal intraepithelial neoplasia.